Chronic Obstructive Pulmonary Disease: A Forgotten Killer

Introducing Health Sciences: A Case Study Approach

Series editor: Basiro Davey

Seven case studies on major topics in global public health are the subject of this multidisciplinary series of books, each with its own animations, videos and learning activities on DVD. They focus on: access to clean water in an overcrowded and polluted world; the integration of psychological and biological approaches to pain; alcohol consumption and its effects on the body; the science, risks and benefits of mammography screening for early breast cancer; chronic lung disease due to smoke pollution – a forgotten cause of millions of deaths worldwide; traffic-related injuries, tissue repair and recovery; and the causes and consequences of visual impairment in developed and developing countries. Each topic integrates biology, chemistry, physics and psychology with health statistics and social studies to illuminate the causes of disease and disability, their impacts on individuals and societies and the science underlying common treatments. These case studies will be of value to anyone who is, or wants to be, working in a health-related occupation where scientific knowledge could enhance your prospects. If you have a wide-ranging interest in human sciences and want to learn more about global health issues and statistics, how the body works and the scientific rationale for screening procedures and treatments, this series is for you.

Titles in this series

Chronic Obstructive Pulmonary Disease: A Forgotten Killer

Edited by Carol Midgley

 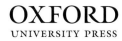

The Open University

OXFORD
UNIVERSITY PRESS

Published by Oxford University Press, Great Clarendon Street, Oxford OX2 6DP
in association with The Open University, Walton Hall, Milton Keynes MK7 6AA.

 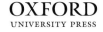

OXFORD
UNIVERSITY PRESS

Oxford University Press is a department of the University of Oxford. It furthers the University's
objective of excellence in research, scholarship, and education by publishing worldwide in

Oxford New York

Auckland Cape Town Dar es Salaam Hong Kong Karachi Kuala Lumpur Madrid Melbourne
Mexico City Nairobi New Delhi Shanghai Taipei Toronto

with offices in

Argentina Austria Brazil Chile Czech Republic France Greece Guatemala Hungary
Italy Japan Poland Portugal Singapore South Korea Switzerland
Thailand Turkey Ukraine Vietnam

Oxford is a registered trade mark of Oxford University Press in the UK and in certain
other countries.

Published in the United States by Oxford University Press Inc., New York

First published 2008. Reprinted 2010

Edited and designed by The Open University.

Typeset by SR Nova Pvt. Ltd, Bangalore, India.

Printed and bound in the United Kingdom by Latimer Trend & Company Ltd, Plymouth.

This book forms part of the Open University course SDK125 *Introducing Health Sciences: A Case
Study Approach*. Details of this and other Open University courses can be obtained from the Student
Registration and Enquiry Service, The Open University, PO Box 197, Milton Keynes MK7 6BJ,
United Kingdom:
tel. +44 (0)870 333 4340, email general-enquiries@open.ac.uk.

http://www.open.ac.uk

British Library Cataloguing in Publication Data available on request

Library of Congress Cataloging in Publication Data available on request

ISBN 9780 1992 3732 6

10 9 8 7 6 5 4 3 2 1

1.2

The paper used in this
publication contains pulp
sourced from forests
independently certified to the
Forest Stewardship Council
(FSC) principles and criteria.
Chain of custody certification
allows the pulp from these
forests to be tracked to the end
use (see www.fsc.org).

ABOUT THIS BOOK

This book and the accompanying material on DVD present the fifth case study in a series of seven, under the collective title *Introducing Health Sciences: A Case Study Approach*. Together they form an Open University (OU) course for students beginning the first year of an undergraduate programme in Health Sciences. Each case study has also been designed to 'stand alone' for readers studying it in isolation from the rest of the course, either as part of an educational programme at another institution, or for general interest and self-directed study.

Chronic Obstructive Pulmonary Disease: A Forgotten Killer is a multidisciplinary introduction to a chronic respiratory condition that has become increasingly common as a result of tobacco smoking or following long-term exposure to smoke or dust pollution. We have included aspects of the biology, chemistry, psychology and epidemiology of the topic, and discuss the impact of modern human living environments and lifestyle choices. No previous experience of studying science has been assumed and new concepts and specialist terminology are explained with examples and illustrations. There is some mathematical content: the emphasis is mainly on interpreting data in tables and graphs, but the text also introduces you step-by-step to some ways of performing calculations that are commonly used in science.

To help you plan your study of this material, we have included a number of 'icons' in the margin to indicate different types of activity which have been included to help you develop and practise particular skills. This icon indicates when to undertake an activity on the accompanying DVD. You will need to 'run' the DVD programs on your computer because they are *interactive*, and this function doesn't operate on a domestic DVD-player. The DVD presents five activities: the first is a video that gives an insight into some personal experiences of chronic obstructive pulmonary disease (COPD); the second and third are guided activities introducing the biology of the respiratory system and the effects of COPD; the fourth is a video showing a visit to a respiratory clinic to see lung function tests in action, and the fifth examines a multidisciplinary approach to supporting people with COPD.

Activities involving pencil-and-paper exercises are indicated by this icon , and if you need a calculator you will see . Some additional activities for Open University students only are described in a *Companion* text, which is not available outside the OU course. These are indicated by this icon in the margin. Some activities involve using the internet and are marked by this icon . References to activities for OU students are given in the margins of the book and should not interrupt your concentration if you are not studying it as part of an OU course.

At various points in the book, you will find 'boxed' material of two types: Explanation Boxes and Enrichment Boxes. The Explanation Boxes contain basic concepts explained in the kind of detail that someone who is completely new to the health sciences is likely to want. The Enrichment Boxes contain extension material, included for added interest, particularly if you already have some knowledge of basic science. If you are studying this book as part of an OU course, you should note that the Explanation Boxes contain material that is *essential* to your learning and which therefore may be *assessed*. However, the content of the Enrichment Boxes will *not* be tested in the course assessments.

The authors' intention is to bring you into the subject, develop confidence through activities and guidance, and provide a stepping stone into further study. The most important terms appear in **bold** font in the text at the point where they are first defined, and these terms are also in bold in the index at the end of the book. Understanding of the meaning and uses of the bold terms is essential (i.e. assessable) if you are an OU student.

Active engagement with the material throughout this book is encouraged by numerous 'in text' questions, indicated by a diamond symbol (◆), followed immediately by our suggested answers. It is good practice always to cover the answer and attempt your own response to the question before reading ours. At the end of each chapter, there is a summary of the key points and a list of the main learning outcomes, followed by self-assessment questions to enable you to test your own learning. The answers to these questions are at the back of the book. The great majority of the learning outcomes should be achievable by anyone who has studied this book and its DVD material; one or two learning outcomes for some chapters are only achievable by OU students who have completed the *Companion* activities, and these are clearly identified.

Internet database (ROUTES)

A large amount of valuable information is available via the internet. To help OU students and other readers of books in this series to access good quality sites without having to search for hours, the OU has developed a collection of internet resources on a searchable database called ROUTES. All websites included in the database are selected by academic staff or subject-specialist librarians. The content of each website is evaluated to ensure that it is accurate, well presented and regularly updated. A description is included for each of the resources.

The website address for ROUTES is: http://routes.open.ac.uk/

Entering the Open University course code 'SDK125' in the search box will retrieve all the resources that have been recommended for this book. Alternatively, if you want to search for any resources on a particular subject, type in the words which best describe the subject you are interested in (for example, 'lung disease'), or browse the alphabetical list of subjects.

Authors' acknowledgements

As ever in The Open University, this book and DVD combine the efforts of many people with specialist skills and knowledge in different disciplines. The principal authors were Carol Midgley (biology), Basiro Davey (pubic health), Lesley Smart (chemistry), Bundy Mackintosh (psychology) and Tom Heller (health and social care). Our contributions have been shaped and immeasurably enriched by the OU course team who helped us to plan the content and made numerous comments and suggestions for improvements as the material progressed through several drafts. It would be impossible to thank everyone personally, but we would like to acknowledge the help and support of academic colleagues who have contributed to this book (in alphabetical order of discipline):

Paul Gabbott, Nicolette Habgood, Hilary MacQueen, Heather McLannahan, James Phillips (biology), Jeanne Katz (health and social care), Elizabeth Parvin (physics), Frederick Toates (psychology) and Kevin McConway (statistics). The media developers who contributed directly to the production of the audiovisual and multimedia components of the DVD were Owen Horn, Jo Mack, Howard Davies, Steve Best, Greg Black and Brian Richardson.

We are indebted to many people who contributed with great enthusiasm and patience to the audiovisual component of this book including: The Breazers group, Joan Higgs (Specialist Nurse), and the staff of The Blue Ball public house, Wharncliffe Side, Sheffield; Dr Rod Lawson (Respiratory Consultant), Dr David Fishwick (Honorary Respiratory Consultant and Chief Medical Officer at the Health and Safety Laboratory), and the staff and patients of the Respiratory Function Unit of the Royal Hallamshire Hospital, Sheffield; Cath O'Connor and the staff and patients attending pulmonary rehabilitation sessions at the Foxhill Medical Centre, Sheffield; and Dr Jim Wild and Dr Neil Woodhouse, Academic Unit of Radiology, School of Medicine and Biomedical Sciences, University of Sheffield.

We would also like to thank Dr Stewart Fisher (Consultant Lung Clinician), Milton Keynes Hospital for critical reading of the manuscript and our External Assessor, Professor Susan Standring (Head of the Department of Anatomy and Human Sciences), Kings College London, whose detailed comments have contributed to the structure and content of the book and kept the needs of our intended readership to the fore.

Special thanks are due to all those involved in the OU production process, chief among them Joy Wilson and Dawn Partner, our wonderful Course Manager and Course Team Assistant, whose commitment, efficiency and unflagging good humour were at the heart of the endeavour. We also warmly acknowledge the contributions of our editor, Bina Sharma, whose skill has improved every aspect of this book; Steve Best, our graphic artist, who developed and drew all the diagrams; Sarah Hofton and Chris Hough, our graphic designers, who devised the page designs and layouts; and Martin Keeling, who carried out picture research and rights clearance. The media project managers were Judith Pickering and James Davies.

For the copublication process, we would especially like to thank Jonathan Crowe of Oxford University Press and, from within The Open University, Christianne Bailey (Media Developer, Copublishing). As is the custom, any small errors or shortcomings that have slipped in (despite our collective best efforts) remain the responsibility of the authors. We would be pleased to receive feedback on the book (favourable or otherwise). Please write to the address below.

Dr Basiro Davey, SDK125 Course Team Chair

Department of Biological Sciences
The Open University
Walton Hall
Milton Keynes
MK7 6AA
United Kingdom

Environmental statement

Paper and board used in this publication is FSC certified.

Forestry Stewardship Council (FSC) is an independent certification, which certifies that the virgin pulp used to make the paper/board comes from traceable and sustainable sources from well-managed forests.

CONTENTS

The DVD activities associated with this book were written, designed and developed by Steve Best, Greg Black, Howard Davies, Owen Horn, Jo Mack, Carol Midgley and Brian Richardson.

CHAPTER I

THE IMPACT OF COPD

Think of an occasion where you have struggled to breathe. Perhaps you have woken at night with a blocked nose during a cold, or found yourself gasping for air after running for a train or a bus? You may recall the desperate urge to get air into your lungs, or the weakness in your limbs. Imagine then, what it might be like to have **chronic obstructive pulmonary disease (COPD)** in which the lungs no longer function efficiently so that breathing becomes a permanent struggle.

COPD is a very common disease, and although you may not have heard of it by this name, you have probably heard of its two main component diseases: *emphysema* and *chronic bronchitis*. COPD is a result of damage to the lungs caused by long-term exposure to inhaled particles of smoke, dust, or fibres and sometimes noxious gases. This may lead you to assume that it is confined to people who work in dusty, heavy industries such as mining or textile manufacture. However, despite the fact that these industries have declined in developed countries such as the UK and the USA, COPD **prevalence** (the total number of people who have the disease at a particular point in time) has continued to increase. Table 1.1 (overleaf) gives some clues why. It shows the impact of leading global health risk factors (Box 1.1) in terms of **disability adjusted life years** or **DALYs** (pronounced 'dailies'). DALYs aim to reflect the real impact of a disease or disability on people's lives. Their calculation is complex but in essence they reflect the total amount of healthy life lost from the combination of premature mortality and years lived with disability or illness. It isn't necessary for you to remember the data in the tables in this book, just the trends that they reveal.

Pulmonary (pronounced 'pul-mon-ar-ee') is a medical term meaning 'of the lungs'. **Chronic conditions** have a gradual onset and are long-lasting. COPD is sometimes referred to by other names including: chronic obstructive respiratory (CORD), airways (COAD), or lung (COLD) disease.

Box 1.1 (Explanation) Risk and risk factors

Risk is the possibility of suffering harm or loss. A health or disease **risk factor** is anything that is *associated* in a population with an increased risk of developing ill health or a particular disease. That is, when the prevalence of a disease is examined in different populations it is found to occur more frequently in those who have been exposed to a certain risk factor than those who have not, or whose exposure level has been lower. However, some people who are exposed to the disease risk factor will *not* develop the disease and some who are not exposed *will*, so the association can only be demonstrated in the *population*, not the individual. It is impossible to predict whether an individual's exposure to a particular risk factor will affect their chance of developing the disease later in life.

Table 1.1 A comparison of the ten leading risks to health in 2000 for the world and for two of the World Health Organization (WHO) regions, Europe and Africa. The per cent (%) contribution of each risk factor to the total disease burden of the region is shown in DALYs. (Source: world data: Rodgers et al., 2004, Table 1, p. 46; Europe and Africa data: WHO, 2002a, Annex Table 12, p. 228)

Rank for health risk factor	WORLD		EUROPE		AFRICA	
	Specific risk factor	% of total DALYs	Specific risk factor	% of region's total DALYs	Specific risk factor	% of region's total DALYs
1	underweight	9.5	high blood pressure	12.8	unsafe sex	11.2
2	unsafe sex	6.3	tobacco smoking	12.3	underweight	4.7
3	high blood pressure	4.4	alcohol	10.1	deficient water supply and sanitation	3.7
4	tobacco smoking	4.1	high cholesterol	8.7	vitamin A deficiency	3.6
5	alcohol	4.0	overweight	7.8	zinc deficiency	3.6
6	deficient water supply and sanitation	3.7	low fruit and vegetable intake	4.4	indoor smoke from cooking fires	3.6
7	high cholesterol	2.8	physical inactivity	3.5	iron deficiency anaemia	3.3
8	indoor smoke from cooking fires	2.6	illicit drugs	1.5	alcohol	2.9
9	iron deficiency anaemia	2.4	lead exposure	0.8	high blood pressure	2.4
10	overweight	2.3	unsafe sex	0.7	lack of contraception	2.1

◆ Use Table 1.1 to identify the sources of exposure to dust, smoke or gases that have a major impact on health.

◆ In developed regions such as Europe, tobacco smoking is the main source of inhaled smoke particles that cause ill health. In developing regions such as Africa (Box 1.2), a more important source is indoor smoke pollution from the burning of solid fuels for cooking and heating (Figure 1.1).

Box 1.2 (Explanation) Classification of country development status

To help simplify the analysis of global patterns of health and disease, countries are often categorised into broad groups by their development status. Several different methods of defining development status are used, combining various indicators such as wealth, education, health, life expectancy, infrastructure, and industrialisation. All methods have the same problem of oversimplifying the situation, often masking important differences between countries within the same group, or between individuals within the same country. Broadly speaking, however, 80% of the world's population live in the 100 or so developing countries.

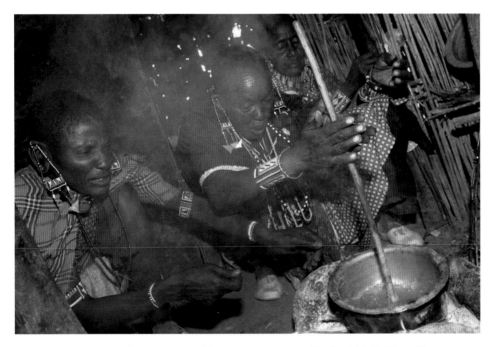

Figure 1.1 Maasai women cooking over an open fire in Rift Valley, Kenya. (Photo: Karen Robinson/Panos Pictures)

1.1 What is COPD?

The lungs occupy most of the space inside the chest and although they appear quite solid they contain a large network of air-filled passages or airways ending in tiny air bags or air sacs (Figure 1.2 overleaf). The lungs are part of the **respiratory system** which transfers oxygen gas from the air into the body, while at the same time expelling the waste gas carbon dioxide that is continuously produced by the body. Long-term exposure to smoke or dust damages the lung airways and air sacs, and may eventually cause COPD. As stated above, people with COPD usually have a combination of two conditions: chronic bronchitis and emphysema. In **chronic bronchitis** (brong-ky-tis) the airways become inflamed and their walls thicken, so that the passage down the middle narrows (Figure 1.2). The damaged airways also produce a lot of thick, sticky mucus which causes frequent coughing. In **emphysema** (em-fuh-see-ma) the walls of the air sacs break down (Figure 1.2) and the lungs become floppy and less elastic, affecting their ability to transfer

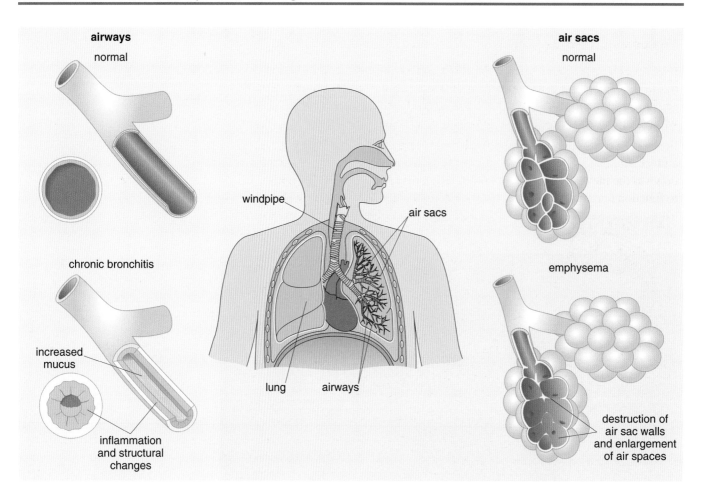

Figure 1.2   The lungs are filled with a network of airways and air sacs. In COPD, damage to the lungs results in narrowing of the airways and destruction of the walls of the air sacs.

gases into and out of the body. The combination of these two conditions obstructs airflow through the lungs and the individual becomes increasingly breathless and fatigued, sometimes to a level requiring confinement to a wheelchair. The damage caused to the lungs is *irreversible*, and the condition is *progressive*; that is, the damage gradually accumulates and the symptoms worsen.

Throughout this book you will find stories or 'vignettes' about two fictitious individuals. These will draw your attention to the problems that people with COPD face in different parts of the world. Vignette 1.1 introduces Jenny.

In the next chapter, some of the risk factors that increase the likelihood of developing COPD are explored, and Chapters 3 and 4, with the help of animations on the accompanying DVD, explain how breathing delivers essential oxygen to the body and how, without it, the body lacks the energy to function. Chapter 5 examines the current theory that the damage to the lungs in COPD results from the body's own attempts to clear away inhaled particles and to protect the delicate airways. In Chapter 6, you will learn about, and observe on the DVD, the types of tests that Jenny took to investigate her lung function. Jenny is experiencing some typical symptoms of COPD: fatigue, breathlessness, wheezing, and a chronic cough that brings up sputum. Certain conditions

Vignette 1.1 Jenny's story

Jenny was born in the 1950s in a small industrial town just north of Manchester in the UK. She took up smoking at an early age. Despite her 'smoker's cough' she has never really considered giving up cigarette smoking which she enjoys while relaxing and socialising with friends and family (Figure 1.3).

For several years she has been aware that her breathing was becoming wheezy and laboured and that her ability to keep active has declined. She has put this down to the inevitable and acceptable effects of ageing, since she has been able to function reasonably well by limiting her daily activities. She is now, however, finding it increasingly difficult to hide the fact that there is something wrong with her breathing. She is breathless most of the time, and has recently given up her part time job at a bakery because it was getting too much for her. Each winter she gets a series of quite nasty chest infections that seem difficult to clear up. On these occasions her breathing can become so difficult that she feels she is suffocating and becomes distressed. Even when she doesn't have a chest infection, her persistent cough affects her almost

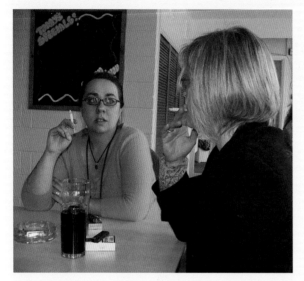

Figure 1.3 Smoking is regarded as an enjoyable social activity by many people worldwide. (Source: Carol Midgley)

every day and produces **sputum** (spew-tum), matter that is coughed up from the lungs and airways and is composed of **mucus** (a viscous secretion produced by the linings of the nose, throat and lungs), mixed with saliva. Her family have noticed that it takes her a long time to get up the stairs, and when she gets to the landing she has to hold on to the banister for a few minutes to recover. On her 53rd birthday she was unable to blow out more than a few candles on her cake, and felt too fatigued to pick up her two-year-old grandson during her birthday party. Upset and embarrassed she has decided to seek professional help and has made an appointment with her local GP. Jenny's GP suspects that she has COPD and arranges for her to have some tests to measure her lung function. He advises Jenny to cut down on her smoking immediately.

such as lung infections or high levels of atmospheric pollution, can result in *exacerbations* of COPD; these are periods of worsened breathing problems. If Jenny has COPD, these exacerbations may become life-threatening and require repeated visits to hospital for breathing assistance. There is currently no cure and no way to reverse the damage to the lungs, but Chapters 7 and 8 will look at how the condition can be managed successfully, and the hopes for improved prevention and treatment in the future. Activity 1.1 looks first at some personal experiences of people with COPD.

Activity 1.1   Living with COPD

Allow 30 minutes

Now would be the ideal time to study the video entitled: 'Living with COPD' on the DVD associated with this book. It was made with the help of 'Breazers', a support and social group attended by people with COPD and other respiratory diseases in Sheffield in the UK. In the film, several people discuss how COPD affects them personally. This activity is an opportunity for you to develop the skill of extracting information from personal *narratives* (stories), and of making notes that you can use at a later date. Make a list of the limitations that COPD imposes on the lives of these individuals. In Chapter 7, we will ask you to reflect on your observations. If you are unable to study the video now, continue with the rest of the chapter and return to it as soon as you can.

1.2   COPD is debilitating and life-threatening

As the symptoms of COPD progress, they can eventually become life-threatening, and patients in the advanced stages are likely to die as a result of complete respiratory system failure or heart failure. In 2002, COPD was the fifth leading cause of death globally and caused many more deaths than all lung and other respiratory system cancers combined. Table 1.2 shows the leading causes of **mortality** (deaths) globally in 2002 compared with a prediction for 2030. We have added arrows to indicate the trends for COPD and diabetes, both of which are expected to contribute an increased proportion of all deaths worldwide by 2030.

◆ Fill in the rest of the arrows yourself to indicate the trends for each of the other conditions. Compare those diseases that are predicted to move further down the table by 2030 with those that are predicted to move up. What types of disease form the bulk of each of these two groups?

◆ Most of the diseases that are predicted to drop *down* the table are infectious or parasitic diseases, including respiratory infections, diarrhoeal diseases, tuberculosis and malaria. An exception is HIV/AIDS. Those diseases that are predicted to move *up* or remain high in the table are mainly non-communicable, chronic conditions such as COPD, cancers, hypertensive disease and diabetes.

There has been progress in controlling infectious and parasitic diseases in many parts of the world through vaccination, antibiotics and improvements in sanitation and living conditions. However, mortality *worldwide* continues to remain high or to increase for non-communicable chronic conditions.

Increasing mortality is only part of the impact of COPD. As you saw in Activity 1.1, COPD imposes a long-term burden of ill health and disability, also known as **morbidity**. In 2002, COPD was the 11th leading cause globally of DALYs (which take into account both morbidity and premature mortality), and according to current projections it will rise to the fourth leading cause by 2030. Nevertheless COPD is often still not recognised as a major public health problem and receives less recognition, less publicity and less

Table 1.2 The leading causes of mortality globally in 2002, and the predictions for 2030. (Source: data in columns 1–3: Murray and Lopez, 1997, p. 124; columns 4–6: Mathers and Loncar, 2006, supplementary dataset S1)

	2002			2030		
Cause of death	No. of deaths (millions)	Rank in 2002	Rank in 2030	No. of deaths (millions)	Cause of death
all causes combined	57.03			73.25	all causes combined
ischaemic heart disease (due to blocked coronary arteries)	7.21	1	1	9.84	ischaemic heart disease
cerebrovascular disease (strokes)	5.51	2	2	7.79	cerebrovascular disease
lower respiratory infections (deep in the lungs)	3.88	3	3	6.50	HIV/AIDS
HIV/AIDS	2.78	4	4	5.68	COPD
COPD	2.75	5	5	2.62	lower respiratory infections
perinatal conditions (affecting babies in the first seven days)	2.46	6	6	2.24	trachea, bronchus and lung cancers
diarrhoeal diseases	1.80	7	7	2.21	diabetes
tuberculosis (without HIV infection)	1.57	8	8	2.11	road traffic accidents
malaria	1.27	9	9	1.58	perinatal conditions
trachea, bronchus and lung cancers	1.24	10	10	1.39	stomach cancer
road traffic accidents	1.20	11	11	1.34	hypertensive disease
diabetes	0.99	12	12	1.15	self-inflicted injuries
hypertensive disease (due to high blood pressure)	0.91	*	*	0.90	diarrhoeal diseases
self-inflicted injuries	0.87	*	*	0.64	malaria
stomach cancer	0.85	*	*	0.62	tuberculosis

* Indicates ranking below the top 12 causes of death.

funding for research and treatment than other illnesses, such as cancers, which affect similar numbers of people. At the end of the book, we will reflect on the question of why societies seem to have been failing to recognise and tackle the issues surrounding this 'forgotten killer'.

One reason may be that the many different names and definitions that have been given to the symptoms of COPD (Mannino, 2002) have made it difficult to determine exactly how many people are affected by the disease, and why. In the next chapter, you will learn about methods that have been used to estimate the prevalence of COPD and also to identify some of the risk factors that determine who is likely to develop the disease.

Summary of Chapter 1

1.1 COPD is a chronic condition that results in breathing difficulties and fatigue, affecting the individual's mobility, ability to function and quality of life. It is ranked fifth worldwide as a cause of mortality and is predicted to increase in the future.

1.2 COPD is a result of gradual damage to the lungs caused by long-term exposure to inhaled smoke, dust, fibres or noxious gases. The damage is irreversible and progressive.

1.3 COPD is a combination of chronic bronchitis (narrowing of the airways, increased production of sputum and a persistent cough) and emphysema (damage to the air sacs that makes the lungs floppy and less elastic and affects their ability to move air in and out of the body).

1.4 Exacerbations of COPD symptoms may require repeated periods in hospital and the advanced stages of COPD are life-threatening, often resulting in respiratory or heart failure.

Learning outcomes for Chapter 1

After studying this chapter and its associated activities, you should be able to:

LO 1.1 Define and use in context, or recognise definitions and applications of, each of the terms printed in **bold** in the text. (Question 1.1)

LO 1.2 Outline the main cause and symptoms of COPD. (Question 1.1)

LO 1.3 Interpret data on the global importance of COPD. (Question 1.2)

LO 1.4 Identify how COPD affects the lives of people in the Breazers group in Sheffield. (DVD Activity 1.1)

LO 1.5 Make notes identifying relevant information from verbal narratives. (DVD Activity 1.1)

Self-assessment questions for Chapter 1

You have had an opportunity to demonstrate LOs 1.4 and 1.5 in DVD Activity 1.1.

Question 1.1 (LOs 1.1 and 1.2)

Explain why COPD is termed a progressive and chronic condition.

Question 1.2 (LO 1.3)

In Table 1.2, what percentage of all deaths globally is predicted to be attributable to COPD in 2030?

WHO GETS COPD?

What exactly is the worldwide prevalence of COPD? It's an important question, because the prevalence of a disease often determines its allocation of the available public health funds and resources. At the moment, it is difficult to give an accurate answer, but there is good reason to believe that worldwide COPD prevalence is underestimated, and that it receives far less attention than it merits in terms of its effects on human mortality, morbidity and quality of life.

2.1 Estimating COPD prevalence

The WHO Global Burden of Disease (GBD) Study collects worldwide data on an annual basis about many different aspects of health and disease. The GBD study estimated that in 2002 the prevalence of COPD in the global population was about 1% or approximately 60 million people (1% of 6 billion).

◆ In Figure 2.1, what is the prevalence rate of COPD in the regions with the highest and lowest levels, and globally how do females compare with males?

◆ The Americas have the highest rate at just less than 16 per 1000 people affected by COPD, while the African region has the lowest at about 2 per 1000 people. Males have a higher prevalence than females globally.

The GBD study collects data from a range of surveys that use different ways of defining and reporting COPD. Many developing countries don't have a centralised health service that collects extensive data about diseases and in these cases the GBD study has to substitute estimates based on countries with similar health profiles. It is suspected that the GBD estimates shown in Figure 2.1 may underestimate COPD prevalence in many world regions because of inconsistencies and inaccuracies in the different ways of collecting data. We will look at one example of a study that has compared different methods of estimating the prevalence of COPD in a

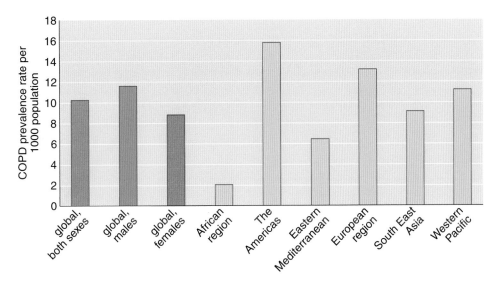

Figure 2.1 A bar chart showing the COPD prevalence rate (per 1000 population) for each of the six WHO world regions, and globally for males and females and both sexes combined. (Source: WHO, 2002b)

randomly selected group of people. The Platino study (Menezes et al., 2005) was carried out in five Central and South American cities (Figure 2.2): Santiago (Chile), São Paulo (Brazil), Mexico City (Mexico), Montevideo (Uruguay) and Caracas (Venezuela). Table 2.1 shows estimates of COPD prevalence from the part of the survey that was carried out in Santiago in Chile.

The participants were asked to complete a questionnaire giving their age, gender, ethnic origin, years of formal education, smoking habits, childhood respiratory problems, and previous exposure to different types of smoke or dust. Then three

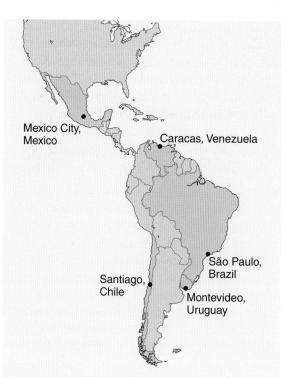

Figure 2.2 A map of Central and South America showing the cities where people took part in the Platino study.

Table 2.1 COPD prevalence (as percentage of survey participants) determined using different methods of diagnosis in Santiago, Chile. (Source: data from Menezes and Victora, 2005, Table 11, p. 25)

Survey participants*	Patient-reported symptoms			Previous doctor's diagnosis			Lung function test	
	Persistent chronic coughing	Breathlessness	Wheezing	COPD	Chronic bronchitis	Emphysema	GOLD guidelines‡	ERS guidelines§
All	6.9%	55.2%	35.0%	1.6%	4.3%	1.6%	6.3%	13.0%
Male	6.7%	42.2%	37.0%	0.9%	2.8%	1.9%	7.5%	17.6%
Female	7.0%	63.3%	33.8%	2.0%	5.3%	1.4%	5.6%	10.2%
Total number of participants	1208	1175	1208	1207	1208	1208	1173	1173

* Participants were aged 40 years or over.
‡ GOLD is the Global Initiative for Chronic Obstructive Lung Disease.
§ ERS is the European Respiratory Society.

different methods of assessing the prevalence of COPD among the people in the study were used:

1   Participants were asked to 'self-report' if they had recently had any respiratory *symptoms* (chronic cough, breathlessness or wheezing).

2   They were also asked if they had ever been *diagnosed* with COPD, chronic bronchitis or emphysema by a doctor.

3   Finally, they were subjected to a **lung function test** that actually *quantified* (expressed as a number or quantity) how well their lungs were functioning. The researchers used a technique called **spirometry** (spie-rom-met-ree) which measures the rate at which an individual is able to force air out of their lungs. The airflow through the lungs of people with COPD is obstructed by the damage to their lungs, so these individuals will only be able to force air out of their lungs at a *reduced* rate compared with a person with healthy lungs. In Chapter 6, you will see how spirometry testing is carried out.

The participants in the Platino survey were treated with a bronchodilator drug (Section 7.2.2) before spirometry tests were carried out to make sure their airways were not temporarily restricted by other conditions such as asthma.

Several national and international organisations that promote respiratory health each have their own guidelines defining a 'healthy' airflow rate. People who fall below this are likely to have COPD. The last two columns of Table 2.1 show different estimates of COPD prevalence using exactly the same spirometry measurements, but following advice from two different health organisations to choose the cut-off level of airflow rate for a COPD diagnosis. GOLD is an organisation called the Global Initiative for Chronic Obstructive Lung Disease. ERS is the European Respiratory Society.

◈   In Table 2.1, about twice as many people (13.0% compared with 6.3%) were diagnosed with COPD on the basis of lung function tests using the ERS guidelines than were diagnosed using the GOLD guidelines. What does this say about the relative 'cut-off' levels for a COPD diagnosis advised by these two organisations?

◆   The airflow rate below which a diagnosis of COPD is made must be set at a higher level in the ERS guidelines because more of the participants have fallen below it and therefore been diagnosed with COPD.

2.1.1 Measuring COPD

As you can see from Table 2.1, the estimates of COPD prevalence in the study population vary enormously depending on the method chosen to define COPD.

◈   Look at Table 2.1 and decide which methods of assessing the prevalence of COPD gave the highest and the lowest estimates.

◆   Self-reported symptoms of wheezing and breathlessness gave the highest estimates of prevalence (up to 55% of all participants). A previous doctor's medical diagnosis of COPD or emphysema gave the lowest estimate (as low as 1.6% of all participants).

Symptoms such as wheezing and breathlessness can occur in many conditions including asthma and mild chest infections or just lack of fitness, so they are likely to give an *overestimate* of COPD prevalence. Conversely, relying on patients to visit a doctor for diagnosis may lead to an *underestimate* of the prevalence of COPD, particularly where access to health services is difficult. In the early stages of COPD, people tend not to seek medical advice, assuming that they are just suffering from a 'smoker's cough', the normal effects of ageing, or some minor ailment. Jenny (Vignette 1.1) only visited her doctor once she felt quite ill and her symptoms were severe enough to affect her daily activity. Studies in several countries suggest that less than half of people with COPD have been diagnosed (Mannino, 2002). Also doctors record their diagnosis using different names for the same condition, so it may be necessary to add together diagnoses of COPD, chronic bronchitis and emphysema to get a more accurate picture. Mortality data may also underestimate COPD because the final cause of death is often recorded as respiratory failure or heart failure, not COPD.

So what method could be used to get a more consistent picture of COPD prevalence? The methods of diagnosing COPD described above are subjective; they are affected by bias introduced by the behaviour of participants (or their doctors) and their personal opinions or understanding of the symptoms. A more accurate method of diagnosis that might eliminate some of these problems would be an *objective* test of lung function based on a *measurable* phenomenon. The Platino study used such a test, by measuring the rate of airflow through the lungs and comparing it with the ideal airflow rate predicted for a healthy individual. As long as the same method of measurement and the same rules for defining COPD are always used, the results should be comparable between individuals in a study, and also between different studies in different parts of the world.

> Objectivity in science involves making judgments that are based on real, demonstrable evidence and that are not influenced by personal feelings, opinions, interpretations, or prejudices.

The GOLD guidelines are currently being promoted as a global standard for diagnosing COPD by lung airflow measurements using spirometry (these will be discussed in more detail in Chapter 6). Using the GOLD guidelines, the Santiago Platino study estimated that about 6.3% of the study participants had low lung airflow levels indicating that they have moderate or severe COPD. It can be assumed that if the participants of the survey are representative of the whole population, a similar proportion of the entire population of Santiago will be affected by COPD. Similar studies using spirometry in several other countries have indicated that between 4 and 10% of their populations are affected by moderate or severe COPD (Halbert et al., 2003).

◆ How does this compare with the GBD estimates of COPD prevalence shown in Figure 2.1?

◆ The prevalence of COPD estimated by these spirometry studies appears to be generally higher than the 2002 GBD estimates.

The limited number of spirometry studies carried out so far may therefore have identified people with COPD who would have been missed in studies that used other methods of collecting data. However, this very much depends on the decision about the 'cut-off' point for a diagnosis of COPD by lung airflow measurements, and there is still some debate about this. Additionally, lung airflow reduction is not exclusive to COPD. So, as you will see in Chapter 6, to make a diagnosis doctors will also consider the complete medical history of the patient, taking into consideration the presence of the COPD risk factors that are discussed below.

2.2 COPD risk factors

The Platino study used the data collected from the questionnaire to look at the association between COPD and particular characteristics of the population, including their ages, occupations and exposure to health risk factors such as tobacco smoking. Table 2.2 shows some of the *variables*, or individual characteristics of the participants, in the Santiago study.

Table 2.2 The relationship between some of the variable characteristics of the study population and prevalence of COPD in the Santiago Platino study, shown as the percentage of each group diagnosed with COPD by lung airflow measurement using the GOLD criteria. (Source: data from Menezes and Victora, 2005, Tables 14 and 15, pp. 30–31)

Variable		% with COPD (GOLD criteria)
Gender:	All	6.3
	Men	7.5
	Women	5.6
Age (years):	40–49	2.8
	50–59	4.0
	>59‡	12.0
Smoking exposure (pack years*):	0	5.4
	<1	3.8
	1–10	3.4
	>10	10.0
Education (years):	0–2	12.8
	3–4	10.3
	5–8	7.1
	>8	4.3

* A pack year is equal to smoking one 20-cigarette pack a day for a year (see text for details).
‡ The symbol > indicates 'more than'; the symbol < indicates 'less than'.

◆ From Table 2.2, what can you say about the relationship between COPD prevalence and the ages of the participants in the Santiago Platino survey?

◆ There is an increase in prevalence with increasing age: fewer people in the lower age groups have COPD than in the higher age groups.

The overall prevalence of COPD in the Santiago Platino study population (using the GOLD criteria) was 6.3%, but for the population aged over 59 years it was almost twice as prevalent (12%). This reflects the fact that COPD develops slowly and progressively as the result of many years of exposure to smoke or dust. The prevalence of COPD is lowest in people less than 40 years of age. This age group were not included in the Platino study, but another study in countries in the European Community indicated that approximately 3% of participants in the 22–44 age range had mild to moderate COPD by the GOLD criteria (de Marco et al., 2004). Because the prevalence of COPD has a strong relationship or *correlation* with increasing age, it is necessary to take into consideration the effects of differences in age structure when comparing different populations. For example, countries with a high percentage of older residents, including many European countries, may apparently have a higher overall COPD prevalence compared with countries with younger populations, e.g. many countries in Africa. The COPD prevalence data collected for each city in the Platino study were therefore *age standardised* by taking a 'standard' or 'reference' population (in this case, that of the whole world population) and using its age structure as a basis for adjusting the populations of the different cities. This enables the data to be directly compared, and the effects of risk factors other than age to be seen more clearly.

2.2.1 Tobacco smoking

The Santiago Platino study also showed that COPD was more prevalent among participants who had smoked the highest quantity of cigarettes; more than 10 pack years (Table 2.2). However, participants who smoked fewer than 10 pack years did not show a higher prevalence of COPD than non-smokers.

◆ Does this mean that participants who had smoked less than 10 pack years had no lung damage?

◆ No, it means that they did not have a sufficient reduction in lung airflow rate to warrant a diagnosis of COPD using the GOLD criteria.

They may however still have had some reduction in lung airflow rate, and since the lung damage caused by smoking is cumulative, some of them may eventually have developed COPD. 5.4% of non-smokers also had COPD, but it is not clear why more non-smokers than low pack year smokers had COPD in this study.

Several studies in both developed and developing countries, including the USA and China, have shown that COPD is most prevalent in populations with high levels of tobacco smoking (Zhang and Cai, 2003). In many countries, tobacco smoking is estimated to account for over 80% of COPD cases and the promotion of schemes to help people stop smoking is now a key element of COPD prevention. Until recently, COPD was regarded predominantly as a male disease because COPD rates tended to be higher for men than women. Many social and cultural traditions discourage women from smoking and from working in dusty, smoky industries. In developed countries, including the UK and the USA,

A pack year is equal to smoking one 20-cigarette pack a day for a year. Four pack years would be four packs a day for a year or one pack a day for four years. Calculating the number of total pack years overcomes the problem of comparing differences in the duration and intensity of smoking.

smoking was rare among women in the early 20th century, but women started cigarette smoking in the 1930s and 40s and the number of women smokers had begun to catch up with the men by the 1960s. This has been reflected in the rapid increase in COPD mortality for women.

Figure 2.3 compares the rates of female and male mortality from COPD between 1968 and 1998 in the USA. Female deaths from COPD increased from about 8 per 100 000 women in 1968 to about 40 per 100 000 of the population in 1998. That's an increase of 400% (divide the increase in the death rate (that's 40 minus 8, or 32, per 100 000) by the starting rate (8 per 100 000) and work out the result as a percentage: $(32 \div 8) \times 100\% = 400\%$).

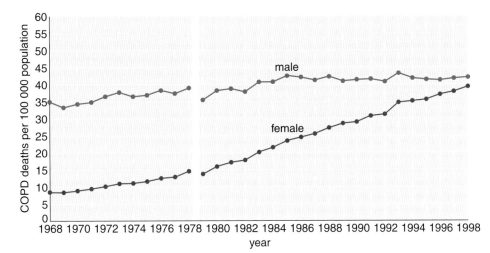
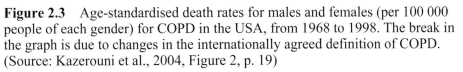

Figure 2.3   Age-standardised death rates for males and females (per 100 000 people of each gender) for COPD in the USA, from 1968 to 1998. The break in the graph is due to changes in the internationally agreed definition of COPD. (Source: Kazerouni et al., 2004, Figure 2, p. 19)

◈   In Figure 2.3, what was the percentage increase in the *male* death rate from COPD between 1968 and 1998?

◆   The male death rate increased from about 35 per 100 000 men to about 42 per 100 000; that's an increase of 7 per 100 000. So $(7 \div 35) \times 100\%$ gives an increase in death rate of 20%.

The COPD death rate for females in the USA has therefore gradually become equal to that of males, probably mainly as result of the large increase in the popularity of cigarette smoking among women. Why did so many women take up smoking (Vignette 2.1)?

Vignette 2.1 Social smoking

Jenny was popular and a trendsetter at school. She became a fan of a local pop group as a teenager in the early 1960s and went to their performances and to parties and social events where both young men and young women smoked cigarettes. At first, Jenny resisted the temptation to smoke and didn't really like the taste or find it very attractive. Eventually Jenny did take up smoking.

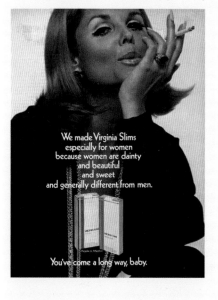

We made Virginia Slims especially for women because women are dainty and beautiful and sweet and generally different from men.

You've come a long way, baby.

◆ Why do you think smoking might have become an established part of her daily activities?

◆ Jenny's peer group may well have exerted pressure on her to share their experience of having a cigarette. Over time, she would have come to associate smoking with fun, relaxation, sexual attractiveness, gregariousness, sophistication and peer approval. Women have also long associated smoking with staying slim. Once Jenny had begun smoking regularly, the addictive nature of tobacco smoking would have made it difficult for her to stop (Box 2.1).

The association of smoking with 'success' would have been reinforced by films, magazines and advertising, which have always used seductive images of emancipation, sophistication, and sexual allure to encourage women to smoke (Figure 2.4), particularly in countries where female roles had begun to change and women aspired to achieve independence.

Figure 2.4   The Virginia Slims cigarette brand was introduced in 1968 in the USA and directly marketed to young, professional women, under the famous slogan, 'You've come a long way, baby.' Some media commentators considered the marketing campaign to be responsible for a rapid increase in smoking among teenage girls. (Source: The Advertising Archives)

Box 2.1 (Enrichment) What's in cigarette smoke?

Cigarette smoke (Figure 2.5) contains thousands of components, the most abundant of which are nicotine, tar and carbon monoxide. Nicotine is the addictive agent that gets smokers 'hooked'. Inhaled nicotine reaches the brain within 15 seconds where it causes the release of dopamine and endorphins, natural chemicals that stimulate the brain, giving a sensation of well-being and decreased anxiety. Nicotine levels remain high in the brain for a couple of hours but then reduce, after which uncomfortable withdrawal symptoms set up cravings for another cigarette. Nicotine itself is not the cause of smoking-related health problems. It is the accompanying tar and toxic gases that cause respiratory diseases and lung cancer. Tar is a dark sticky substance formed from smoke particles mixed with water vapour. It also contains hundreds of chemicals including *toxins* (poisonous substances) and *carcinogens* (cancer-causing chemicals).

Carbon monoxide is a toxic gas that is also found in car exhaust fumes and other types of smoke pollution. Carbon monoxide binds to haemoglobin, the oxygen-transporting complex found in the blood, preventing it from carrying oxygen around the body (Chapter 4).
Numerous other toxic gases are mixed with the smoke, including ammonia, formaldehyde, and hydrogen cyanide. Some of these have irritant properties and some are known or suspected carcinogens.

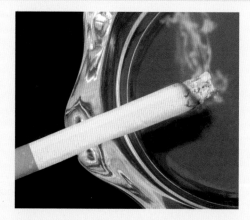

Figure 2.5   The particles in cigarette smoke and tar, together with irritating gases and toxic chemicals, are responsible for lung damage and COPD in many smokers. (Source: Arturo Delfin/Morguefile)

As long as cigarette smoking remains normal and acceptable behaviour in adults, discouraging children and adolescents from smoking is difficult. The governments of most developed countries are taking measures to reduce incentives to smoke, but while smoking prevalence is levelling off in the developed world, it is increasing in developing nations where there are fewer government controls and much less public debate about the adverse effects of tobacco. By the mid-2020s, the WHO predicts that 85% of all smokers will come from the world's poorest countries (Figure 2.6), where governments can ill afford to support the health costs involved, and smoking-related diseases will become the world's major killer. Many developing countries hesitate to restrict tobacco use, fearing that they might lose foreign investment. Some, including Brazil, India and China, are also tobacco growers and exporters, making them even more reluctant to adopt stricter controls and lose a valuable cash crop.

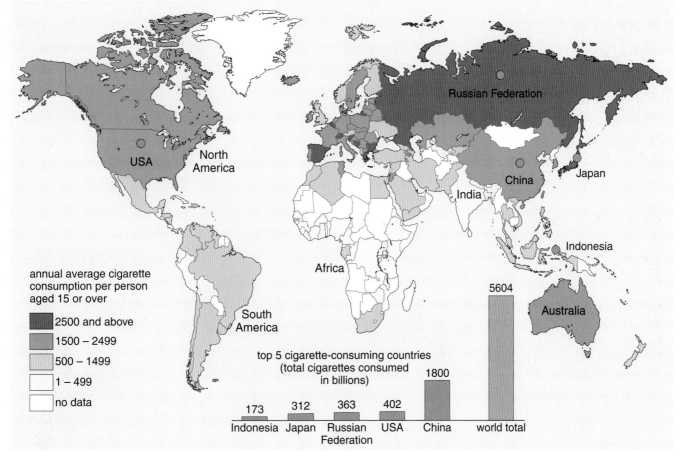

Figure 2.6   A map of worldwide annual average cigarette consumption per person aged 15 years or over in 2004 or using latest available data, and total cigarettes consumed in the top five countries. (Source: Adapted from Mackay et al., 2006, p. 32)

2.2.2 Occupational exposure to smoke or dust

You can probably think of many situations where people are exposed to high levels of smoke, dust or fumes as part of their daily work. There are few studies about how many of the world's workers are affected by COPD, but prevalence has been reported to be higher in several occupations including coal and mineral mining, metal grinding and welding, farming and grain-handling, construction work, transport and the manufacture of textiles, paper, chemicals, rubber, plastics and food (Hnizdo et al., 2002).

◈ Could occupational exposure have contributed to Jenny's condition (look back at Vignette 1.1)?

◆ She had previously worked part time in a bakery where exposure to flour dust could have added to the total amount of dust particles she inhaled.

It is estimated that approximately 15% of COPD cases globally may be attributable to occupational exposure (Boschetto et al., 2006). However, disentangling the effects from those of tobacco smoking can be difficult. People who work in smoky, dusty occupations, particularly male-dominated industries, are also more likely to be tobacco smokers. To estimate the *attributable risk*, i.e. the proportion of the total risk that is contributed by an individual risk factor, it is necessary to compare disease prevalence in exposed and non-exposed groups. Where there are multiple COPD risk factors involved this becomes very complex.

In the UK, coal-workers are the only occupational group for whom extensive statistics about the COPD risk attributable to occupational dust exposure have been collected. This is reflected in the fact that compensation was made available for coal-workers with emphysema and chronic bronchitis under the UK government's industrial injuries scheme in 1993. Workers in many other industries have not been offered similar compensation schemes due to the lack of sufficiently robust evidence linking occupational exposures to development of COPD. Nevertheless, the governments of most developed countries have increasingly imposed health and safety procedures that monitor **particulates** (fine particles of a solid suspended in the air, Box 2.2) in the environment and minimise the exposure of workers (Figure 2.7), although the standards of safety vary greatly around the world.

Box 2.2 (Explanation) Measuring the level of particulates in the environment

Health and safety legislation in many countries requires that smoky or dusty working environments and areas with heavy traffic or pollution are regularly monitored for the concentrations of toxic gases and small particulates known as PM_{10} (pee-em-ten). These are particles with a diameter of less than 10 μm. Air quality in terms of particulates is often quoted as the PM_{10} concentration in micrograms per cubic metre (written scientifically as μg m^{-3}). These tiny particles are able to pass into the lungs, causing inflammation and disease. They are usually a mixture of smoke, soot, dust, and the products of chemical reactions undergone by the pollutants emitted by motor vehicles and industrial processes.

μm is the abbreviation for micrometre. There are 1 000 000 or 10^6 μm in a metre. m^3 is an abbreviation for a cubic metre, the volume of a cube with edges one metre in length, and m^{-3} means per cubic metre.

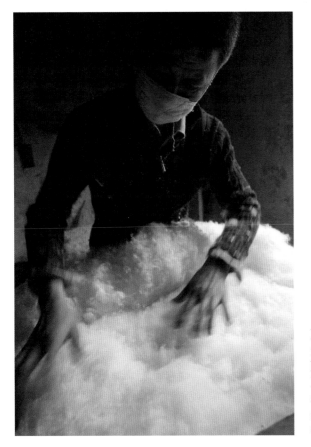

Figure 2.7 Cotton-worker in Chongqing, China, handling a bale of raw cotton. Large amounts of cotton dust and fibres are released at this stage of processing. (Source: China Photos/Getty Images)

2.2.3 Indoor smoke pollution

In many developing countries, there are high levels of COPD even when tobacco smoking is rare (Bruce et al., 2002). Clean fuels (Figure 2.8 overleaf) for cooking and heating, particularly electricity, are expensive and half of the world's population (around 3 billion people) instead rely on coal, an impure fossil fuel extracted from the ground by mining, or **biomass fuels** derived from plant material or animal waste (including wood, dried animal dung, crop residues or charcoal). Many people are therefore regularly exposed to very high levels of indoor smoke (Vignette 2.2 overleaf).

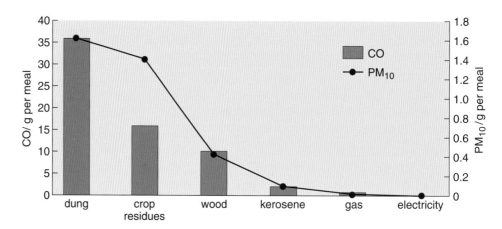

Figure 2.8   The energy ladder is a scale that rates the quality of household fuel, shown here as output of grams (g) of PM_{10} and carbon monoxide gas during preparation of an average meal. The dirtiest are traditional biomass fuels, while gas fuels are the cleanest for burning. Cooking with electricity is too costly for poor households. (Source: Warwick and Doig, 2004, Figure 8, p. 14)

Vignette 2.2   Nadira's family

Nadira is a 48-year-old mother of five children living in an extended family with her husband Musafir, his elderly parents and one aunt in a remote rural community in Badakhshan Province, northeastern Afghanistan. The family house is built from local stones and is roofed with beams interwoven with branches. The focus of family life is the tandoor oven (Figure 2.9) and the raised platform around it on which the family eats and sleeps.

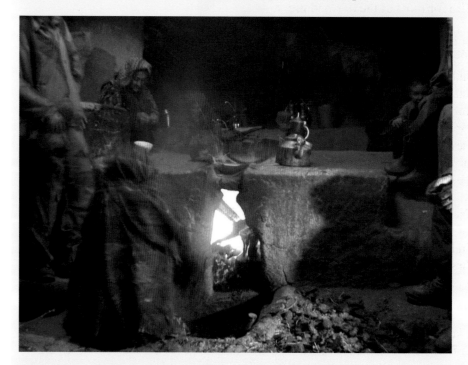

Figure 2.9   Afghan women cooking with a traditional tandoor oven are exposed to smoke and airborne ash. (Source: Alex Duncan)

The oven is surrounded by a pit where Nadira stands while she is cooking and into which she rakes the ashes from the open fire. In the mountainous region in which she lives, Nadira builds fires from corn husks, branches and dried dung from the family's goats and yak. Smoke from the fire rises through the house and exits through a hole in the brushwood roof. At times, the smoke inside is so dense that it is hard to breathe, but it has a practical value as a repellent for the blood-sucking parasites that drop down from the roof at night.

◆ Which members of this household do you think will have the most exposure to indoor smoke pollution and why?

◆ Nadira, the younger children and the elderly adults spend longer periods in the house (and inhaling smoke from the fire) than Musafir and the older children, who are outside more of the time tending animals and crops, gathering fuel and collecting water. Nadira has the highest exposure of all because she has to lean into the smoke as she tends the fire and cooks the family meals.

The indoor concentration of PM_{10} particles (Box 2.2) in dwellings such as this one, averaged over a 24-hour period, is typically between 300 and 3000 $\mu g\ m^{-3}$ of air, but it may reach 10 times this level during cooking (Bruce et al., 2000). The safe exposure limit for PM_{10} recommended by the US Environmental Protection Agency is 150 $\mu g\ m^{-3}$. Nadira and the other members of her family are exposed to high concentrations of particulates and harmful gases such as carbon monoxide for many hours a day throughout their lives. In the long hard winters, they are inhaling smoke from the indoor fire for most of the day and night.

It is very rare for women in Afghanistan to smoke tobacco; adult men in rural communities generally smoke using a hookah, sometimes referred to as a hubble-bubble pipe, which filters tobacco smoke through water before it is inhaled. Despite the difference in their smoking habits, the levels of chronic respiratory diseases – including COPD – among adults in populations like Nadira's are similar between the sexes throughout rural communities in the developing world. Women typically spend the most time beside the fire and are at the greatest risk of developing COPD as a result of indoor smoke pollution (Ekici et al., 2005; Shrestha and Shrestha, 2005).

Nadira's mother-in-law, Bibi Gul, has difficulty in 'catching her breath' most of the time and cannot exert herself without becoming breathless. Bibi Gul is in her early 60s (she does not know her exact age), but for several years she has been losing her sight as cataracts increasingly cloud the lens in both her eyes. There is growing evidence that absorption into the lens of toxins from smoke may contribute to the development of cataracts (Pokhrel et al., 2005).

Cataracts are explained in another book in this series, *Visual Impairment: A Global View* (McLannahan, 2008).

Nadira's five children have all suffered repeated episodes of **lower respiratory infections** (which affect the lungs, including pneumonia, see Table 1.2) and several studies have shown that these infections occur more often among young children exposed to indoor smoke (Smith et al., 2000).

The importance of clean water and adequate sanitation are explored in another book in this series, *Water and Health in an Overcrowded World* (Halliday and Davey, 2007).

The WHO estimates that about 22% of COPD globally is caused by exposure to indoor smoke, and around 1.6 million people die every year as a result of all indoor smoke-related illnesses combined (Figure 2.10), including about a million children – almost as many as are killed by unsafe water and poor sanitation. 80% of these deaths occur in rural communities such as Nadira's in poor countries all over the world.

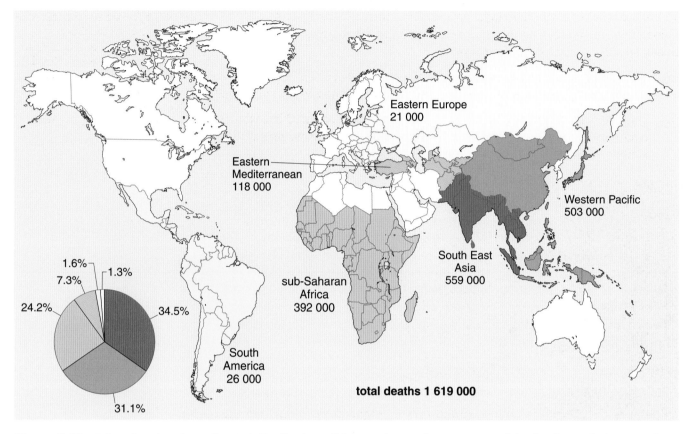

Figure 2.10 Map showing the estimated distribution of the number and percentage of deaths due to indoor smoke from solid fuels in the most affected regions in 2000. These are deaths from several conditions, not just COPD. (Source: Warwick and Doig, 2004, Figure 3, p. 5)

Much of the work to try to reduce ill health due to indoor air pollution is carried out by charities and non-governmental organisations. One of these, 'Practical Action' (originally called ITDG, the Intermediate Technology Development Group), was founded in 1966 by the radical economist Dr E. F. Schumacher to prove that his philosophy of 'small is beautiful' could bring improvements to people's lives through small local projects. Now turn to Activity 2.1.

Activity 2.1   Reducing the effects of indoor smoke pollution

Allow 30 minutes

In this activity, you will visit Practical Action's website to learn about their projects to reduce ill health due to indoor air pollution (Figure 2.11). Go to the 'Practical Action – Indoor air pollution' website which is available through Open University ROUTES (see 'About this book' on p. vi). Spend no more than 15 minutes reading about individual projects that reduce the health effects of indoor air pollution (at the time of writing there were active projects in Kenya, Sudan and Nepal). Use this information to:

(a)   write down *three* suggestions for practical measures that could be used to reduce the effects of indoor smoke on the health of Nadira and her family, and

(b)   suggest *three* difficulties that you envisage may be encountered in enabling, or persuading the family to take up these measures. Comments on this activity are included at the back of this book.

If you are studying this book as part of an Open University course, you can access this website directly via a link from the course website. You should also go to the *Companion* associated with this book for more information and to complete Activity C1.

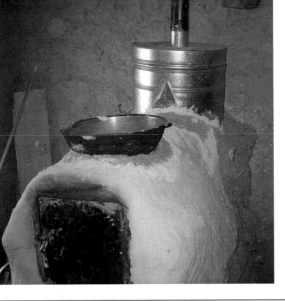

Figure 2.11   A flue attached to a tandoor oven in an Afghan house removes most of the smoke. (Source: Alex Duncan)

Figure 2.12 (overleaf) shows the probability of developing COPD for men and women living in homes in Xuanwei, China, according to whether or not their stove had a chimney. In statistics, the mathematical probability of an event happening is a value that always lies between 0 and 1. An event that is certain to happen is given a probability value of 1. If the probability is 0, then that event will never occur. An event that is equally likely to happen or not happen is given a probability value of 0.5. In Figure 2.12, all men and women were COPD-free at age 24 whether or not they had a chimney, i.e. the probability that they will have COPD is 0. However, as they get older the probability that they will develop COPD increases.

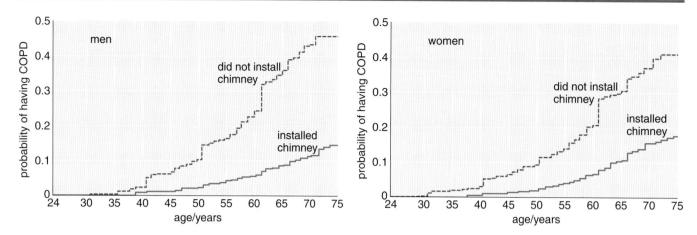

Figure 2.12 Line graphs showing the probability of having COPD by a certain age in men and women in Xuanwei, China, according to whether their stove had a chimney. Data from a survey made between 1976 and 1992. (Source: adapted from Chapman et al., 2005, Figure 1, p. 2)

◆ In Figure 2.12, what is the probability that women will develop COPD by the age of 60 if their stove (a) has a chimney and (b) has no chimney?

◆ The probability for (a) is about 0.06 and for (b) is about 0.2. The probability is increased fourfold in the absence of a chimney.

2.2.4 Outdoor air pollution

Studies from the UK and the USA have shown that high outdoor air pollution levels increase the number of exacerbations (episodes of severe and even life-threatening breathing problems) in people who *already* have respiratory diseases such as COPD and asthma. However, so far there is no strong evidence to prove that outdoor air pollution increases the risk of *developing* respiratory diseases such as COPD, so the role of modern urban pollution remains controversial. Severe air pollution events in the past have, however, demonstrated the dangers of very high levels of smoke pollution. The great London smog of December 1952 was caused by smoke from coal fires mixing with winter fog (Figure 2.13) and is still the worst UK air pollution disaster on record. It lasted for five days and may have caused as many as 12 000 deaths. Most of the people affected probably already suffered from respiratory diseases or heart problems.

As a direct result the British government introduced its first Clean Air Act in 1956 which introduced smokeless zones in urban areas and made grants available to householders to convert their homes from traditional coal fires to heaters fuelled by gas, oil, smokeless coal or electricity. Such severe smogs are a thing of the past in London now that coal use has diminished, but other rapidly industrialising countries are experiencing increasing problems. China is using its huge reserves of coal to run most of its rapidly growing number of power stations because it possesses relatively little petroleum and natural gas.

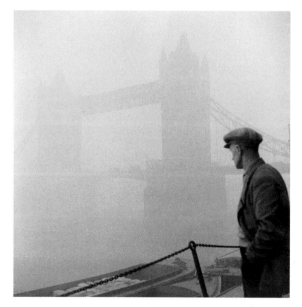

Figure 2.13 The great London smog in December 1952 may have caused 12 000 deaths. (Source: Getty Images)

In recent years, large-scale atmospheric pollution events have also occurred in the form of massive forest fires. In 2005, Malaysia announced a state of emergency in several areas after fires lit to clear land in neighbouring Indonesia seriously reduced air quality and visibility across the Malacca Strait (Figure 2.14). More widespread is the increasing level of pollution from motor vehicles and aeroplanes, particularly in the world's growing megacities (those with populations in excess of 10 million people). Although there is little evidence so far that outdoor air pollution is a significant risk for developing COPD, the accumulation of PM_{10} particles and fumes, including those generated by fires and industrial or vehicle pollution, probably adds to each individual's total burden of respiratory damage.

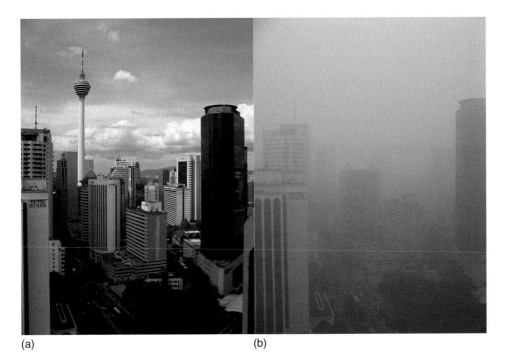

(a) (b)

Figure 2.14 (a) A view of Kuala Lumpur in Malaysia on a clear day. (b) Smoke from forest fires in Indonesia envelops the city. (Source: PA Photos)

2.3 Susceptibility to developing COPD

Exposure to high levels of dust or smoke is not the only factor that determines whether an individual will develop COPD. Only about 25% of people who are lifelong tobacco smokers will go on to develop it (Løkke et al., 2006), although many more will have some degree of impairment of their lung function. Several factors have been proposed to explain why some individuals are more vulnerable than others (Table 2.3), including exposure to early childhood infections or to respiratory allergens that may sensitise the lungs to the damaging effects of particles. Some people may have so-called 'hyper-reactive' airways that are very prone to constriction (narrowing), for example people with asthma (Chapter 6). Dietary deficiencies, problems with lung development during childhood, and inherited genetic make-up (which we will discuss further in Chapter 5) may also

Allergens are substances that may trigger allergic reactions in the lungs, e.g. pollen.

contribute. COPD is a **multifactorial disease**, meaning that a combination of several biological and environmental factors contribute towards its development.

The Santiago Platino study used the number of 'years spent in education' as a very crude marker of social and economic status (Table 2.2) and found that COPD prevalence was highest amongst those people who had experienced the least schooling. There are many reasons why social status might affect COPD risk (Prescott and Vestbo, 1999), for example tobacco smoking and occupational exposures to smoke and dust are higher amongst those people from poorer backgrounds. Poverty also increases exposure to poor housing conditions including dampness, overcrowding and indoor smoke pollution. In some cases, poor nutrition and weight loss can reduce the strength and endurance of the muscles required for lung function. Undernourished mothers give birth to lower-birth-weight babies, and since lung growth is related to processes occurring during fetal growth and childhood development, their offspring may start at a respiratory disadvantage.

Table 2.3 A summary of environmental and biological risk factors that may contribute to the likelihood of developing COPD.

Environmental factors	Biological factors (characteristics of the body)
tobacco smoke	inherited genetic factors (e.g. alpha-1 antitrypsin deficiency which we will discuss in Chapter 5)
occupational dusts, fibres and airborne chemicals	
indoor and outdoor atmospheric pollution	hyper-reactive airways that are prone to constriction
infections and allergens	deficiencies in lung growth associated with fetal or childhood development
socioeconomic circumstances	changes in lung structure during ageing
cultural influences	
dietary deficiencies	

Summary of Chapter 2

2.1   It is currently very difficult to determine accurately the global prevalence of COPD, owing to lack of data and variation in the diagnostic methods used in different studies. The WHO estimates that COPD affects 1% of the world's population, but more recent spirometry studies suggest that the proportion may be higher (between 4 and 10%) in many countries.

2.2   Spirometry is an objective method of diagnosing COPD by measuring lung airflow. The results are comparable between different populations as long as the same method and the same criteria are used for making a diagnosis.

2.3   The damage caused to the lungs is progressive and most individuals only start to experience symptoms in their 50s and 60s. Because age is a major risk factor in the development of COPD, it is necessary to age-standardise data in order to compare different populations with different age distributions.

2.4 The major environmental risk factor for developing COPD is long-term exposure to airborne smoke, fibre or dust particles. In industrialised countries, the main sources are tobacco smoking and occupational exposure, while in the developing world women and children are particularly vulnerable to indoor smoke from cooking fires. The contribution of outdoor pollution to the development of COPD is less clear, but it can make respiratory problems worse and increase respiratory disease-related mortality.

2.5 Reducing exposure to smoke and dust particles, e.g. by fitting stoves with hoods or chimneys to vent smoke out of houses, is an effective way of reducing COPD.

2.6 Not all individuals who experience the same degree of exposure to airborne particles will develop COPD, so other currently less well-defined factors such as genetic inheritance, diet or previous exposure to respiratory infections or allergens may also affect the level of risk.

Learning outcomes for Chapter 2

After studying this chapter and its associated activities, you should be able to:

LO 2.1 Define and use in context, or recognise definitions and applications of, each of the terms printed in **bold** in the text. (Questions 2.1, 2.2 and 2.3)

LO 2.2 Outline some of the different ways that have been used to estimate the prevalence of COPD in a population, and discuss their advantages and disadvantages. (Question 2.1)

LO 2.3 Interpret data on disease prevalence from graphs and tables. (Questions 2.1 and 2.2)

LO 2.4 Discuss the different types of risk factors that contribute to the development of COPD. (Questions 2.2 and 2.3)

LO 2.5 Use examples to discuss the sources of smoke and dust particle pollution that are associated with COPD around the world, and ways in which exposure can be reduced. (Question 2.3 and DVD Activity 2.1)

LO 2.6 Extract information from an internet website. (DVD Activity 2.1)

If you are studying this book as part of an Open University course, you should also be able to:

LO 2.7 Evaluate the validity and reliability of information obtained from a website. (Activity C1 in the *Companion*)

Self-assessment questions for Chapter 2

You have also had the opportunity to demonstrate LOs 2.5 and 2.6 in DVD Activity 2.1.

Question 2.1 (LOs 2.1, 2.2 and 2.3)

Explain why, in Table 2.1, lung-function testing by spirometry indicates that there may be a higher prevalence of COPD in the population than is indicated by the number of people who are diagnosed with COPD by a doctor.

Question 2.2 (LOs 2.1, 2.3 and 2.4)

Look at Figure 2.1 and give one possible reason why the WHO estimate of the COPD prevalence rate in Africa is much lower than for Europe.

Question 2.3 (LOs 2.1, 2.4 and 2.5)

Identify two human activities that may increase an individual's risk of developing COPD, and in each case give an example of a country or region of the world where you think each activity is likely to be a major risk factor, giving reasons for your choices.

CHAPTER 3

THE RESPIRATORY SYSTEM

The respiratory system (the lungs and other structures involved in exchanging gases with the environment) and the **cardiovascular system** (the heart and the blood circulation) work together to deliver oxygen, a gas present in the air, to all parts of the body. The mechanisms that drive these processes are involuntary; that is, you do not normally apply any conscious thought to maintaining them. When one part of them fails, however, there are wide-reaching consequences.

3.1 The role of oxygen in the body

In the next two chapters we will look at why the body needs oxygen (Figure 3.1), and what happens if the delivery system begins to break down as it does in COPD. First it may help to summarise some of the scientific conventions used to describe molecules and their interactions (Box 3.1).

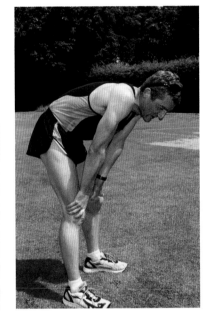

Figure 3.1 Intense exercise has depleted oxygen from this athlete's body and left him gasping for air. (Source: Mike Levers/Open University)

Chemical structures and reactions are discussed in more detail in two other books in this series (Halliday and Davey, 2007; and Smart, *Alcohol and Human Health*, 2007).

> **Box 3.1** (Explanation) Elements, atoms and molecules
>
> All types of matter are made up of **elements**. An element is a substance that cannot be broken down into a simpler substance; it is composed of **atoms**. For example, hydrogen gas is made up of hydrogen atoms and oxygen gas is made up of oxygen atoms. An atom is the smallest unit of matter that is capable of taking part in a chemical reaction. Each element has been assigned a chemical symbol, usually the first letter or two from its name. For example:
>
> - the symbol for carbon is C
> - the symbol for oxygen is O
> - the symbol for hydrogen is H.
>
> **Molecules** are formed when two or more atoms join together by forming chemical bonds. The atoms of each element form a characteristic number of bonds with other atoms. Hydrogen atoms can only form one bond, oxygen usually forms two. A molecule of hydrogen gas is formed when a single bond is made between two hydrogen atoms:
>
> single bond
> H—H
>
> A molecule of oxygen gas is formed by a double bond (represented by a double line) between two oxygen atoms :
>
> double bond
> O=O
>
> Oxygen can bond with two hydrogen atoms simultaneously through two single bonds to form water.
>
> H—O—H
>
> Carbon usually forms four bonds, and can form double bonds with two atoms of oxygen to give carbon dioxide:
>
> O=C=O

A sugar molecule such as glucose is somewhat larger:

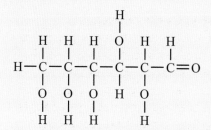

The representations above, known as **structural formulae**, are useful for understanding the structure of these simple molecules but are time-consuming to write down, so to simplify things, chemists have developed a chemical short-hand for representing molecules. These **chemical formulae** tell us which type of atoms a molecule contains, and a subscript number after the element symbol indicates when there is more than one of a particular type of atom.

For example, water is represented as H_2O, showing that it contains two hydrogen atoms and one oxygen atom; oxygen gas, represented by O_2, contains two oxygen atoms and carbon dioxide gas is CO_2.

◆ How many of each type of atom does a single glucose molecule contain?

◆ Glucose contains 6 carbon, 12 hydrogen and 6 oxygen atoms.

Conventionally the chemical formula for glucose is written down as: $C_6H_{12}O_6$.

In reality most molecules are not flat and linear as they appear in a structural formula but adopt complex 3-dimensional structures.

Cells are the basic structural and functional units of organisms. Some organisms, such as bacteria, are single-celled; others, such as humans, are multicellular.

Most people interpret the term **respiration** to mean breathing, and indeed the human lungs and other structures involved in breathing are referred to as the respiratory system. However, the term 'respiration' has a second meaning: the chemical reactions that take place in the individual cells of all organisms to release energy from nutrients. To reduce confusion, we will refer to this latter process as **cellular respiration**. The most efficient form of cellular respiration requires oxygen. A fire requires oxygen to burn fuel, releasing energy as heat and light. Similarly, in cellular respiration, oxygen is used to break down glucose (and other high-energy sugars and fats derived from food) releasing *chemical energy*. The reaction of molecules with oxygen is called **oxidation**. The chemical energy released is required to power cellular processes, for example the contraction of muscle cells during body movement, or the manufacture of proteins by all types of cell (Box 3.2). Equation 3.1 shows the chemical representation of the oxidation of glucose ($C_6H_{12}O_6$) to release chemical energy:

chemical energy release

$$6O_2 + C_6H_{12}O_6 = 6CO_2 + 6H_2O \qquad (3.1)$$

Box 3.2 (Explanation) Proteins are very large molecules

Although the structural formula of glucose looks complicated, it is a relatively simple molecule compared with many others found in the bodies of organisms. Some of these are made up of many hundreds or thousands of atoms, and are too complex to write down even as chemical formulae. The largest group of these are the **proteins**. These are composed mainly of the elements carbon, hydrogen, oxygen and nitrogen (chemical symbol, N) and are long chain-like molecules built up from smaller molecules called *amino acids*. The protein chains fold up into complex shapes necessary for their widely varying functions in the body's cells and tissues. Examples of proteins are **enzymes**, which speed up (*catalyse*) chemical reactions such as glucose oxidation. Many other proteins have a structural role in maintaining the shape of cells and tissues.

Six molecules of oxygen and one molecule of glucose (the *reactants*) react to form six molecules of carbon dioxide ($6CO_2$) and 6 molecules of water ($6H_2O$) (the *products*).

◈ In Equation 3.1, how many atoms of carbon, oxygen and hydrogen are there in total in the reactants and how many in the products of the reaction?

◆ There are, in total, 6 carbon, 18 oxygen and 12 hydrogen atoms in both the reactants and in the products.

So this is a *balanced equation*; that is, all of the atoms in the reactants are incorporated into the new products of the reaction (oxygen and glucose are converted into carbon dioxide and water).

We should point out here that this is a great simplification of what happens in a cell. In fact, if the oxidation process happened in this single one-step reaction, the cell would 'burn up' on releasing the energy. The reaction actually takes place in several complex steps involving protein enzymes (Box 3.2). These steps gradually release energy from nutrients in a chemical form that cells can store for use in other types of chemical reaction.

Cells contain the equivalent of small 'engines' called **mitochondria** (migh-toe-kon-dree-ah) where cellular respiration takes place, so these need a constant supply of oxygen. Despite the vital importance of oxygen, the human body cannot store it. When deprived of air for more than a few minutes, the lack of chemical energy will prevent essential cell functions, so cells will begin to die. This occurs particularly rapidly in brain cells and unconsciousness and death will rapidly result. A build-up of the waste product of cellular respiration, carbon dioxide, is also harmful to the body, and, as you will see in Chapter 4, it must be removed. Now try Activity 3.1 overleaf.

Balancing chemical equations and the release of chemical energy from molecules are explained in another book in this series (Smart, 2007).

Activity 3.1   Respiration and COPD

Allow 40 minutes

Now would be the ideal time to study the interactive sequence entitled: 'Respiration and COPD' on the DVD associated with this book. This will help you to visualise the processes of breathing and gas exchange, and the consequences of COPD that are described in the next few chapters. There are self-assessment questions throughout the DVD sequence, which you should attempt to answer before pressing the 'answer' button in each case. You can move on to the next section once you are ready, by clicking on the forward arrow button. If you are unable to study this activity now, continue with the rest of the chapter and return to it as soon as you can.

3.2   Oxygen is obtained from the air

Most organisms need a way of exchanging gases with the environment in order to obtain oxygen for cellular respiration, and to expel the waste gas carbon dioxide. Gas exchange is a fairly straightforward process for a single-celled organism such as a bacterium, which simply exchanges gases with its surroundings directly by diffusion through the thin cell membrane that encloses it (Box 3.3).

Humans, as multicellular organisms, have a more complex problem: how to get oxygen to all of the estimated 10^{12} (a million million) individual cells in the human body.

◆ Can you think of a reason why you cannot simply exchange gases through your body surface like a bacterium?

◆ The human body is covered in a protective tissue, the skin, that acts as a barrier, containing and protecting our internal organs and tissues against infection and dehydration. It isn't very permeable to fluids or gases.

Another reason is that the surface area of the body is small in comparison to its volume and by the simple process of diffusion, gases wouldn't penetrate very far into the body. It wouldn't be possible to supply the cells deep inside the body with oxygen. Respiration, in the sense of breathing and gas exchange, is therefore much more complex in multicellular organisms. Human respiration can be divided into five steps:

1   *ventilation* which brings air into the lungs (and expels air containing waste carbon dioxide)

2   *exchange* of respiratory gases between the lungs and the blood

3   *transport* of respiratory gases around the body in the blood

4   *exchange* of respiratory gases between the blood and the body tissues

5   and finally *cellular respiration* which we have already mentioned: the release of chemical energy from nutrient molecules by oxidation in the individual cells of body tissues.

Box 3.3 (Explanation) Diffusion

Molecules in a gas or a liquid constantly move around. They naturally spread out from a region where they are at a relatively high concentration, into areas where they are at a lower concentration. This is the process of **diffusion**, sometimes called passive diffusion (meaning no energy expenditure is required). It will continue until the whole available area has the same concentration of the molecules. A good example of diffusion is the ability of a drop of coloured ink to spread slowly and evenly throughout a glass of water. The same process can also proceed across a thin barrier that is *permeable* to small molecules, i.e. they can pass through it freely. All cells are enclosed by a barrier called a **cell membrane** which is composed of a double layer (a bilayer) of lipid (fatty) molecules (Figure 3.2). It is permeable to very small molecules such as gases, but impermeable to larger molecules. Gases such as oxygen can diffuse across the cell membrane when there is a *concentration gradient*; that is, if the concentration of oxygen is *higher* outside the cell than it is inside, the oxygen molecules will diffuse into the cell. Once the molecules reach an equal concentration on both sides of the membrane, diffusion will cease. The processes we describe in this chapter rely on the diffusion of small molecules across cell membranes, or across the thin walls (composed of a single layer of cells) of lung airways and small blood vessels. In each case, it is the same process: the movement of small molecules from an area where they are at high concentration into an area where they are at a lower concentration.

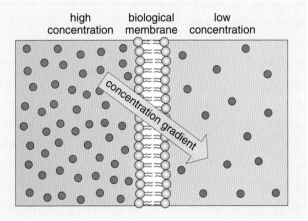

Figure 3.2 Schematic representation of diffusion across a cell membrane.

You will now learn more about steps 1–4 of respiration described on the previous page and how they are affected in people with COPD.

3.2.1 Ventilation of the lungs

Air enters the body through the nose and mouth (Figure 3.3). The linings of the nasal cavity and the larger airways in the lungs produce sticky mucus which

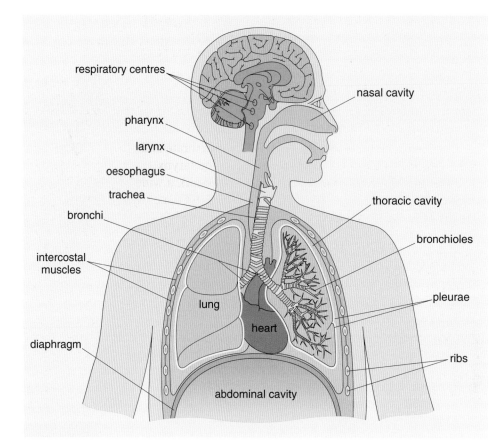

Figure 3.3 The components of the respiratory system. The microstructure of the alveoli and associated blood vessels is shown in greater detail in Figure 3.6.

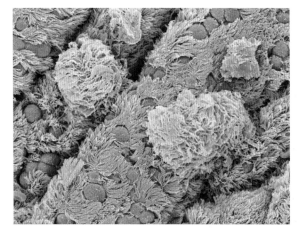

Figure 3.4 An artificially coloured scanning electron microscope picture (magnified to about 2000 times actual size) of mucus-producing cells (round and orange) and hair-like cilia (yellow) lining a bronchus. Mucus drops (pale pink) and a piece of dust (pale green) are also seen. (Source: Susumu Nishinaga/Science Photo Library)

traps many of the particles polluting the air. Small hair-like structures called cilia (silly-ah) on the surface beat back and forth, sweeping the mucus towards the throat where it can be swallowed, or coughed out (Figure 3.4). This helps to prevent particles and micro-organisms or **microbes** such as bacteria, from getting further into the respiratory system. The air passes into the throat or pharynx (fah-rinks), where it is joined by air that has entered through the mouth. There are two openings in the throat, one leading to the oesophagus and the digestive system and the other to the voice box or larynx (lah-rinks) and the rest of the respiratory system.

◈ What normally happens if a piece of food accidentally enters the airways?

◆ There is an irresistible urge to cough.

The presence of food, dust or mucus stimulates the tips of nerves in the lining of the airways causing an involuntary *reflex response*. A small amount of air is taken into the lungs, the larynx closes trapping the inspired air, and muscles in the abdomen (the cavity containing the stomach, intestines and other organs) contract, forcefully pushing the contents of the abdomen up against the muscular **diaphragm** (dye-uh-fram) which separates the chest cavity from the abdominal cavity. The larynx then opens and the air is squeezed out under pressure, producing a cough and clearing the airways. Sneezing is a reflex response to irritation of the nasal passages.

The larynx also contains the vocal folds which vibrate and produce sound as air moves over them. From the larynx, air passes into the windpipe or **trachea** (tra-kee-ah), a wide hollow tube about 2 cm in diameter that is held permanently open by semicircles of a tough **connective tissue** called cartilage (Box 3.4). The trachea divides into two branches called **bronchi** (brong-kye), which serve the left and right lungs. Each bronchus divides into two smaller bronchi which divide again and again, forming a series of increasingly smaller bronchi, and then even smaller **bronchioles** (brong-kee-ohls) that are less than 1 mm in diameter. There are over 1500 miles of airways in the average human lung, forming a shape like an upside-down tree with branches and twigs; which is often actually referred to as the *bronchial tree* (Figure 3.5).

The reflex response, (involuntary muscular activity triggered by stimulation of the nervous system) is described in another book in this series, *Pain* (Toates, 2007).

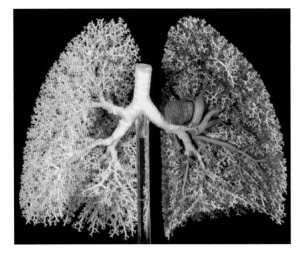

Figure 3.5 A model of the lungs showing the bronchial tree. The airways of the lungs are shown in yellow on the left-hand side of the picture, and the right-hand side shows in addition the associated network of blood vessels coloured blue and red. (Source: Walter Weder)

Box 3.4 (Explanation) Connective tissue

Connective tissues have many different roles in binding together, supporting and protecting other tissues and organs in the body. They are made up of cells embedded in a matrix of fibres formed from protein molecules. The fibres are mainly composed of the proteins *collagen* (coll-ah-jen), which provides strength, or *elastin* (ee-lass-tin) which provides flexibility, although the proportions of the different types of protein fibres vary. Some connective tissues are hard, with densely packed collagen fibres to provide support and strength. Examples are bone, and also cartilage which forms the semicircular rings that hold the trachea open, and provides a smooth surface at the ends of bones where the moving parts of joints slide over each other. There are also soft, loose connective tissues which are composed of more loosely packed protein fibres. Loose connective tissues in the lung contain a high proportion of elastin fibres which help to provide elasticity to the walls of the airways and air sacs.

The estimated surface area of the lung airways and air sacs of an adult human is about 80 m² (an area covered by 80 squares each measuring 1 m x 1 m).

The bronchioles at the tips of the bronchial tree open into tiny air sacs (bag-like structures) called **alveoli** (al-vee-oh-lye, singular: alveolus (al-vee-oh-luss)) that are about 0.2 mm in diameter (Figure 3.6). The walls of the alveoli are only a single-cell thick and are the respiratory surface where oxygen diffuses into the body. Gases, including oxygen, in the air inside the alveoli dissolve in the film of moisture on the surface of the alveolar wall and diffuse across into very small blood vessels called **capillaries** inside the lung tissue (Figure 3.7). The waste gas carbon dioxide can diffuse in the other direction from the pulmonary capillaries into the alveoli so that it can be exhaled (Chapter 4). The entire bronchial tree is closely associated with an equally complex 'tree' of blood capillaries as shown in Figure 3.5, giving a very large contact area between the lungs and the blood circulation where gas molecules can be exchanged.

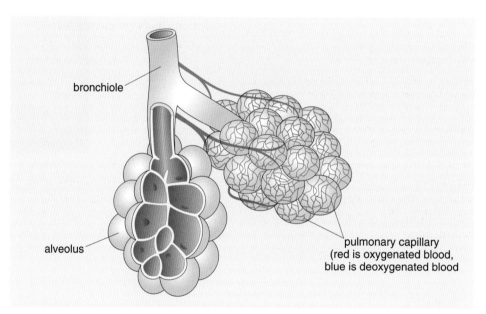

Figure 3.6 A schematic diagram of alveoli in contact with pulmonary (lung) blood capillaries.

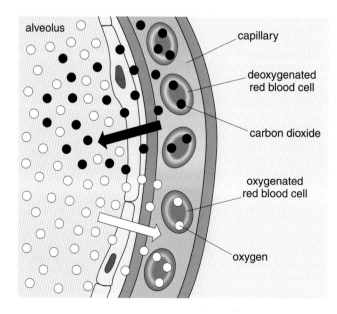

Figure 3.7 A schematic diagram to show the diffusion of gases (oxygen is white, carbon dioxide is black) between an alveolus and a pulmonary blood capillary.

The lungs fill the chest cavity (the thoracic cavity (thor-as-ik)) which is formed between the ribcage and the muscular diaphragm (Figure 3.8). The lungs are completely enclosed by a bag formed from two thin sheets of tissue called pleurae (ploor-ee). The outer pleura (ploor-uh) is attached to the chest wall, the inner one to the lungs, and the space between them is filled with fluid so that the two pleurae slide against each other. This allows the lungs to move easily during breathing, and prevents the lungs from collapsing by holding them to the chest wall. The lungs act like bellows, drawing air in during inhalation or **inspiration**, and pushing it out during exhalation or **expiration**.

3.2.2 Inspiration

Breathing is usually under the control of the autonomic or involuntary nervous system, the part of the nervous system that maintains body processes that do not require control by the *conscious* mind. The process of breathing starts in **respiratory centres** in a region of the brain called the medulla. These centres send a series of *action potentials* along nerves which stimulate the muscular diaphragm and the muscles between the ribs (the *intercostal* muscles) to contract. When relaxed, the diaphragm is dome-shaped and curves upwards into the thoracic cavity (Figure 3.8). When it contracts during inspiration (breathing in), it flattens out and moves downward. The ribs are attached to the spine and the breast bone (sternum), and contracting the muscles between them moves the ribcage upwards and outwards. These movements increase the volume of the chest cavity, and the lungs, which are effectively stuck to the chest wall by the pleurae, also expand to fill the space and air flows in. Before reading about why this happens, you should first read Box 3.5 (overleaf) which explains the significance of gas pressure.

An action potential is a change in electrical charge in a nerve that occurs when it is stimulated. Another book in this series (Toates, 2007) explores how signals are transmitted by action potentials.

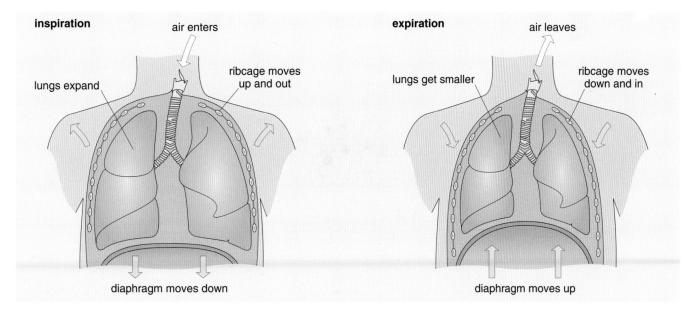

Figure 3.8 During inspiration, the chest cavity increases in volume as the diaphragm and the muscles between the ribs contract. During expiration, the relaxation of the diaphragm and muscles reduces the volume and the air flows out again.

Box 3.5 (Explanation) Gas pressure

Imagine a balloon full of oxygen gas. The oxygen molecules are constantly moving around and collide with each other, and with the surface of the balloon, so that there are many thousands of billions of collisions each second. The force of impact of a single collision is too small to be measured; however, taken all together, the huge total number of impacts exerts a force on the inner surface of the balloon so that it keeps its inflated shape and volume. This collective force is the **gas pressure**. If you were to squash the sealed balloon to reduce its size and its volume, the oxygen molecules would be more crowded together, or compressed, there would be a larger number of molecular collisions, and the gas pressure would be higher (even though the balloon contains the same *number* of oxygen molecules as before). Gas molecules always move from a region of high pressure (a high concentration of gas molecules) into a region where there is lower pressure (a lower concentration of gas molecules), until the pressure is even throughout. This happens rather suddenly when you pop a balloon.

The measurement of gas pressure for different purposes has resulted in a confusing array of different units of measurement. The standard international (SI) unit for pressure is the pascal (Pa); however, pulmonary physiologists and chest physicians still use an older convention where pressure is expressed in terms of millimetres of mercury (mmHg). Hg is the chemical symbol for mercury (from its Latin name, *hydrargyrum*). An instrument called a manometer is often used to measure differences in pressure (Figure 3.9) and consists of a U-tube containing a column of liquid mercury. The height (in millimetres) to which the mercury column is pushed up the U-tube depends on the pressure applied to each end. You may have had your blood pressure measured using a device that works on the same principle, although more modern instruments use very different technology.

If you are curious, 760 mmHg is equal to 101 325 pascals (Pa) or 101.325 kilopascals (kPa).

Air is a mixture of nitrogen, oxygen, water vapour and carbon dioxide, plus a few other gases in very small quantities. The contribution of each individual gas to the overall gas pressure of air is called its **partial pressure**. The total gas pressure of a mixture of gases, such as air, is therefore the *sum* of the partial pressures of all of its constituent gases. The total **atmospheric pressure** of air, i.e. the pressure exerted by all of the gases in the Earth's atmosphere, is 760 mmHg at sea level. Notice that sea level is specified. This is because atmospheric pressure decreases as altitude increases. As you travel higher into the atmosphere there is less air weighing down on the air underneath, so the gas molecules are more spread out (less compressed). Air pressure at sea level is used as the standard atmospheric pressure throughout this book.

◆ Oxygen constitutes about 21% of the air, so what is its partial atmospheric pressure at sea level in mmHg?

◆ Oxygen partial pressure is 160 mmHg (21% of 760 or (21 ÷ 100) × 760 = 160 mmHg).

Partial pressure is denoted in this book by the symbol P, followed by the chemical formula of the gas it relates to, so for example P_{O_2} is used to denote the partial pressure of oxygen.

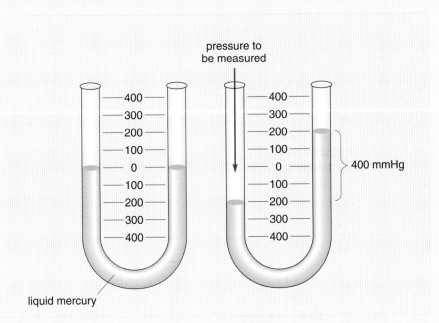

Figure 3.9 Schematic diagram of a manometer. The difference in air pressure on either side of the column of liquid mercury in the tube can be read from the scale as the difference between the heights of the two sides of the column. In this diagram the pressure difference is 400 mmHg.

Figure 3.10 (overleaf) shows a manometer filled with mercury indicating the difference between external atmospheric air pressure, and the air pressure inside the lungs. In resting lungs at the end of expiration, the air pressure in the alveoli and the outside atmosphere is equal as indicated by the equal level of mercury on each side of the manometer (Figure 3.10a). During inspiration (Figure 3.10b) the volume of space inside the lungs increases and the air molecules already inside spread out into the larger area, so that the gas pressure inside the lungs becomes lower than the external atmospheric pressure (the lungs are sometimes said to have *negative pressure* compared with the outside air, although this term is rather misleading). The mercury level is pushed down on the side of the manometer exposed to the atmosphere, and up on the lung side, because the pressure from the atmosphere is now greater than that inside the lungs (Figure 3.10b). Air from outside flows into the lungs until the gas pressure is equalised between the inside and the outside, at which point the flow of air into the lungs ceases and the two sides of the mercury column become level again (Figure 3.10c).

3.2.3 Expiration

As the lungs fill up with air, stretch sensors in the lungs transmit action potentials along nerves to the respiratory centres in the brain informing them that the chest is fully expanded. The respiratory centres stop sending the action potentials

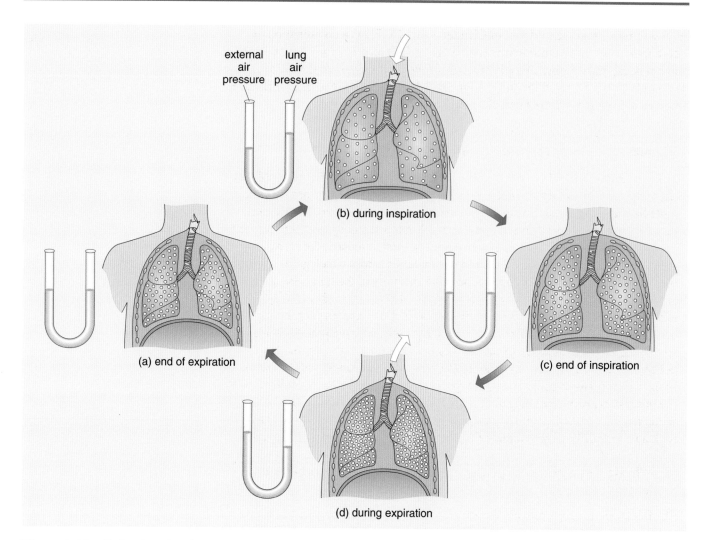

external air pressure   lung air pressure

(b) during inspiration

(a) end of expiration

(c) end of inspiration

(d) during expiration

Figure 3.10   Enlarging the chest cavity draws air into the lungs due to the change in air pressure. The diagram shows the lungs at different stages of inspiration and expiration. In each case a manometer filled with mercury indicates the difference in air pressure between the lungs and the external atmosphere. (a) Resting lungs at the end of expiration. (b) During inspiration. (c) Maximum inspiration. (d) During expiration (see text for details).

that cause the rib muscles and diaphragm to contract, and they relax again. The chest cavity moves back to its former size, releasing the tension on the elastic lungs which spring back or *recoil* to their original smaller size, squeezing and compressing the gas inside the lungs (like the balloon described in Box 3.5) so that the gas pressure becomes higher than the outside atmospheric pressure (Figure 3.10d). The gas inside the lungs therefore flows out until gas pressure equalises with the outside atmosphere. The alveoli of the lungs in fact act rather like tiny balloons – it requires effort (muscle contraction) to inflate them, but when the inflating pressure is released, the recoil of the elastic walls of the alveoli allows them to deflate, like a balloon. Breathing out, or expiration, is therefore a *passive* event. It is simply the result of the relaxation of the diaphragm and rib muscles and the elastic recoil of the lungs.

You will recall that we told you in Chapter 1 that COPD is a combination of two conditions: chronic bronchitis (narrowing of the airways and blockage by thick mucus) and emphysema (destruction of the elastic walls of the alveoli, leaving large airspaces in the lung; Vignette 3.1). Most people with COPD have a mixture of both emphysema and chronic bronchitis.

Vignette 3.1   Jenny's expiration is obstructed

Jenny is finding that whenever she does anything strenuous she **hyperventilates**, i.e. breathes very rapidly and deeply, over-inflating her lungs. She has to work quite hard to push the air out again. She feels very breathless and the effort of breathing is tiring. This is a sign that she has developed emphysema. Destruction of alveolar walls in emphysema has two effects. First, it reduces the area of contact between the alveoli and the blood capillaries across which gases can diffuse (Section 3.2.1). Second, it reduces the elasticity of the lungs. Because Jenny's lungs are floppy and 'compliant', she is able to inflate them easily, even taking in a slightly larger volume of air than normal to overcome her feeling of breathlessness. However, when she expires, her lungs no longer recoil efficiently, so they fail to push out all of the air. In addition, her floppy airways tend to collapse near the end of her expiration, trapping air in the lungs, and her chronic bronchitis and mucus production narrow the airways, which also contributes to the obstruction to the escaping air. Jenny's hyperventilation helps to keeps her blood quite well oxygenated; however, at the end of each expiration she is left with an abnormally large volume of oxygen-depleted air still inside her lungs.

◆ Why do you think this may make Jenny hyperventilate (overinflate her lungs)?

◆ Because her lungs remain abnormally full of 'stale' air at the end of expiration, she has to inflate them much more than normal to obtain enough 'fresh' air.

The breathlessness caused by COPD is therefore mainly due to a mechanical defect that reduces the efficiency of ventilation and the rate at which gases can be exchanged with the environment. It is not so much a problem of getting 'fresh air' in, than of getting 'stale air' out. The extra effort required to breathe is very tiring and can be alarming. The following experiment may give you some idea of what COPD feels like; place a drinking straw in your mouth and hold your nose so that you can only breathe in and out through the straw. How long does it take you to become breathless and open your mouth to breathe freely?

In Chapter 5, we will look at how airborne particles damage the lungs, causing emphysema and chronic bronchitis, but first we will continue to follow the route of oxygen into the body.

3.2.4 Exchange of gases between the lungs and the blood

Inspired air entering the lungs contains oxygen at its atmospheric partial pressure (P_{O_2}) of 160 mmHg, but by the time it reaches right down to the alveoli, the P_{O_2} is actually lower (about 100 mmHg, Figure 3.11) because the newly inspired air has mixed with a residual volume of air that always remains in the lungs and has very little oxygen left in it (Chapter 6). This residual volume is often larger than normal in people with emphysema (Vignette 3.1). Gases in the inspired air, including oxygen, will dissolve in the film of moisture on the alveolar walls and enter the nearby blood capillaries by diffusion.

◆ How does concentration affect the diffusion of gas molecules across an alveolar or a capillary wall?

◆ The molecules move from the side where they are at higher concentration to the side where there is a lower concentration, until there is an equal concentration of the molecules on both sides.

The ability of oxygen to diffuse into the blood is therefore dependent on the fact that the concentration of oxygen in the alveoli following inspiration is higher than its concentration in the blood inside the capillaries (Figure 3.11).

In the next chapter, we will explore how oxygen and carbon dioxide are transported around the body in the blood circulation. Although the gaseous oxygen is now dissolved in the blood, pulmonary physiologists rather confusingly still use gas pressure units (mmHg) to refer to its concentration. Once blood reaches the tissues of the body, oxygen diffuses out into the tissues and is used up by cellular respiration, so the partial pressure of oxygen (P_{O_2}) in the blood circulation drops to 40 mmHg during its journey around the body. The blood then returns to the lungs where oxygen is replenished.

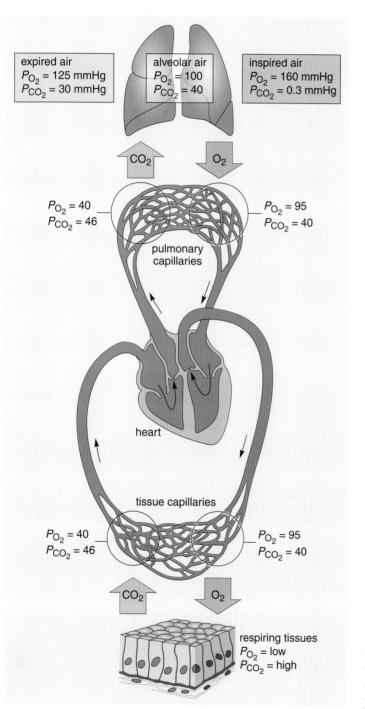

expired air
P_{O_2} = 125 mmHg
P_{CO_2} = 30 mmHg

alveolar air
P_{O_2} = 100
P_{CO_2} = 40

inspired air
P_{O_2} = 160 mmHg
P_{CO_2} = 0.3 mmHg

CO_2 O_2

P_{O_2} = 40
P_{CO_2} = 46

P_{O_2} = 95
P_{CO_2} = 40

pulmonary capillaries

heart

tissue capillaries

P_{O_2} = 40
P_{CO_2} = 46

P_{O_2} = 95
P_{CO_2} = 40

CO_2 O_2

respiring tissues
P_{O_2} = low
P_{CO_2} = high

Figure 3.11 The partial pressures of oxygen and carbon dioxide in the body. Oxygen-rich blood leaving the lungs and travelling to the tissues is shown in red. Oxygen-depleted blood leaving the tissues and travelling to the lungs is shown in blue. Gas pressures of oxygen and carbon dioxide at different stages of the journey are indicated. All pressures are in mmHg.

Summary of Chapter 3

3.1   The cells of the body require oxygen for cellular respiration (the release of chemical energy from high-energy nutrients such as glucose). The energy is required for many cellular processes including muscle contraction. The carbon dioxide produced as a waste product of cellular respiration is toxic and must be expelled from the body.

3.2   Gases such as oxygen and carbon dioxide dissolve in surface moisture and move across cell membranes and the thin walls of the alveoli and blood capillaries by the process of passive diffusion.

3.3   The extensive networks of airways and blood capillaries in the lungs provide a large surface contact area with very thin walls across which large numbers of oxygen and carbon dioxide molecules can diffuse at each breath.

3.4   Breathing is controlled by the autonomic nervous system, the part of the nervous system that maintains body processes that do not require control by the conscious mind. Respiratory centres in the brain send action potentials along nerve cells. These stimulate the diaphragm and rib muscles to contract.

3.5   Active muscular contraction of the diaphragm and ribcage muscles expands the chest cavity and the lungs causing an inspiration of air. Expansion of the lungs creates low gas pressure inside the lungs compared with the outside atmospheric pressure, so air flows in until the gas pressure between the lungs and the outside atmosphere is equalised.

3.6   Oxygen-depleted air is expired *passively* when the muscles relax again. The elastic recoil of the lungs allows them to spring back into shape as the chest cavity reduces in size, pushing out the air.

3.7   In emphysema, the lack of elastic recoil by the lungs prevents efficient expiration and a large residual volume of oxygen-depleted air is trapped in the lungs. People with emphysema tend to hyperventilate (overinflate) their lungs to compensate for this.

Learning outcomes for Chapter 3

After studying this chapter and its associated activities, you should be able to:

LO 3.1   Define and use in context, or recognise definitions and applications of, each of the terms printed in **bold** in the text. (Questions 3.1, 3.2, 3.3 and 3.4)

LO 3.2   Interpret the chemical notation used to write down chemical structures. (Question 3.1)

LO 3.3   Explain where and how oxygen is used in the process that provides the body with energy. (Question 3.1)

LO 3.4   Work out the concentration of gases in terms of gas pressure using the units commonly employed to describe blood gas concentrations. (Question 3.2)

LO 3.5   Describe how ventilation moves air in and out of the lungs, and what role gas pressure plays in this process. (Question 3.3)

LO 3.6   Describe the components of the respiratory system and the structure of the airspaces in the lungs. (Question 3.3 and DVD Activity 3.1)

LO 3.7   Explain how gases can move between the lungs, the blood circulation and the tissues by the process of diffusion. (Question 3.4 and DVD Activity 3.1)

Self-assessment questions for Chapter 3

You have also had the opportunity to demonstrate LOs 3.6 and 3.7, in the self-assessment questions associated with DVD Activity 3.1.

Question 3.1 (LOs 3.1, 3.2 and 3.3)

What molecules are the *products* of the oxidation of glucose? Write them down as molecular formulae.

Question 3.2 (LOs 3.1 and 3.4)

Nitrogen constitutes 78% of air. What is its partial atmospheric pressure at sea level, expressed in mmHg?

Question 3.3 (LOs 3.1, 3.5 and 3.6)

Briefly explain the mechanism that is responsible for the flow of gases *out* of the lungs during expiration.

Question 3.4 (LOs 3.1 and 3.7)

Why aren't the *proteins* inside a cell lost by diffusion out of the cell?

CHAPTER 4

DELIVERING OXYGEN TO THE TISSUES

4.1 Haemoglobin carries oxygen

The oxygen-carrying capacity of blood is facilitated by a carrier molecule called **haemoglobin** (hee-moh-gloh-bin). The red blood cells, which biologists call **erythrocytes** (e-rith-ro-sites), each contain a large number of these complex molecules. Haemoglobin is an assembly of smaller molecules (Figure 4.1): four proteins called *globins*, each folded around a molecule called *haem* (pronounced 'heem'). Each of the four haem molecules holds at its centre an atom of iron (Fe), which is able to form a bond with one oxygen molecule, so that one complete haemoglobin molecule can carry four oxygen molecules at once. Haemoglobin with oxygen bound is called **oxyhaemoglobin**. The iron atoms in haemoglobin are normally derived from the diet but sometimes iron tablets are prescribed for people with anaemia (low haemoglobin levels).

The secret of haemoglobin's ability to transport oxygen to body tissues is that oxygen binds to it *reversibly*. When there are many oxygen molecules present (P_{O_2} is high) in the lungs after an inspiration of air, most of the haemoglobin molecules in the red blood cells (erythrocytes) inside pulmonary (lung) capillaries will become oxyhaemoglobin, carrying four oxygen molecules. Blood containing a large proportion of oxyhaemoglobin is referred to as **oxygenated blood**. When the oxygenated blood circulates into blood capillaries in tissues where the P_{O_2} is very low, the oxyhaemoglobin separates or *dissociates*, into haemoglobin and free oxygen molecules. The oxygen then diffuses into the tissues.

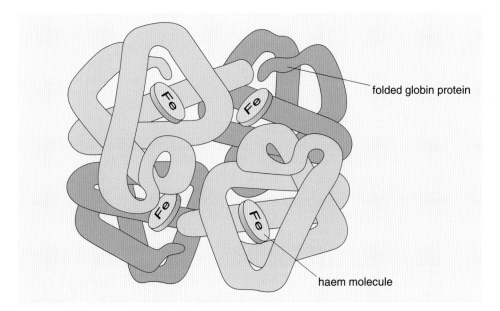

folded globin protein

haem molecule

Figure 4.1 A schematic diagram of haemoglobin. The four yellow 'disks' represent the haem molecules, each containing an iron atom (represented by its chemical symbol, Fe) where the oxygen molecule binds, while the four blue folded 'sausage shapes' represent the globin proteins.

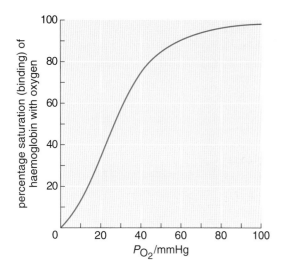

Figure 4.2   An oxygen–haemoglobin dissociation curve shows that haemoglobin binds more oxygen as oxygen partial pressure (P_{O_2}/mmHg) increases.

The reversible binding of oxygen to haemoglobin can be represented using an oxygen–haemoglobin dissociation curve (Figure 4.2). The horizontal axis of the graph shows increasing oxygen partial pressure (P_{O_2}), and the vertical axis shows the percentage of the haemoglobin molecules that are *saturated* with oxygen, i.e. are carrying four oxygen molecules. As the partial pressure of oxygen increases, more haemoglobin molecules bind to oxygen until almost 100% are saturated.

◆ In Figure 4.2, what percentage of haemoglobin molecules is saturated with oxygen at a P_{O_2} of 40 mmHg? (Hint: draw a line up from the horizontal axis to the curve, then another across to the vertical axis to read off the value.)

◆ Approximately 75%.

It is haemoglobin that gives the familiar red colour to blood, and oxygenated blood in the arteries is bright red. Blood that has passed through the tissues and lost some of its oxygen (**deoxygenated blood**) is slightly darker red, although it may appear slightly blue in the veins because of an optical effect caused by the way in which light penetrates through the skin. In diagrams, however, oxygenated blood that has just come from the lungs is conventionally represented by the colour red, and deoxygenated blood that has passed through the tissues and is on its way back to the lungs, by blue.

4.1.1   Carbon monoxide blocks oxygen binding to haemoglobin

The presence of other gases in the blood can affect how well haemoglobin will bind to oxygen molecules. You have already come across the gas carbon monoxide in Chapter 2. Its molecular formula is CO, which doesn't appear to obey the bonding rules (Section 3.1), but since its bonding is complex, we won't go into it here.

◆ Can you recall any sources of carbon monoxide in the air we breathe?

◆ Carbon monoxide is found in smoke pollution including vehicle exhaust fumes, tobacco smoke and smoke from burning biomass fuels.

Carbon monoxide is an extremely toxic gas that binds to the haem part of haemoglobin like oxygen, but it binds *irreversibly*, forming **carboxyhaemoglobin**. Carboxyhaemoglobin can no longer bind to oxygen because the carbon monoxide has permanently occupied the oxygen bonding sites. This reduces the number of haemoglobin molecules in the blood that are available to transport oxygen. Symptoms of carbon monoxide poisoning are nausea, headaches and light-headedness. Prolonged exposure can result in unconsciousness, brain damage and death. Carboxyhaemoglobin is bright pink in colour, so carbon monoxide poisoning makes the skin turn very pink. Several other gases that are found in air pollution, for example hydrogen sulfide (H_2S), can also bond with haemoglobin preventing it from carrying oxygen. New red blood cells and haemoglobin are continuously produced by the body to replace worn out red blood cells, so the body can eventually recover from the effects of these toxic gases.

4.1.2 Hypoxia

A condition where all or part of the body is deprived of oxygen, whether through the effects of low oxygen in the atmosphere, toxic gases such as carbon monoxide, or defects in the respiratory system (Vignette 4.1), is called **hypoxia**.

◆ Can you suggest why climbers are in danger of experiencing hypoxia at very high altitudes?

◆ The partial pressure of oxygen in the atmosphere is lower at high altitude than at sea level (Box 3.5). The oxygen concentration is lower, so the concentration gradient between the atmospheric air and the blood will not be very great. During an inspiration, fewer oxygen molecules will diffuse from the lungs into the blood.

Symptoms of whole-body hypoxia include a blue colouration, called cyanosis (sigh-an-oh-sis), of the skin, the lips and finger nails because deoxygenated blood appears slightly blue under the skin; also headaches, fatigue, shortness of breath, nausea, unsteadiness (Vignette 4.1), and eventually seizures (convulsions due to lack of oxygen in the brain) and coma (prolonged unconsciousness).

Vignette 4.1   Bibi Gul has developed symptoms of advanced COPD

Nadira's mother-in-law Bibi Gul, who you first met in Vignette 2.2, is in her 60s and spends much of her time inside the house keeping an eye on her family. After many years of daily exposure to smoke from the fire, she is having increasing episodes of chronic coughing which produce a lot of sputum, and she has recurrent respiratory infections. Moving around is a big effort for her now, so she spends even more time indoors. She has frequent exacerbations of her symptoms – increased breathlessness, wheeziness, sputum and coughing, and headaches. She frequently feels fatigued, confused, nauseous and sleepy and her skin, particularly her lips, has a slightly blue-ish tone.

◆ Can you suggest any reasons for symptoms such as fatigue, headache and blue skin tone?

◆ Bibi Gul has too little oxygen in her blood and is developing symptoms of hypoxia.

She is suffering from headaches and confusion because her brain cells are being starved of the oxygen required for cellular respiration and her muscle cells don't have enough energy to sustain exercise, so she finds moving around very tiring. Carbon monoxide poisoning may also be contributing to her symptoms by further reducing the oxyhaemoglobin in her blood.

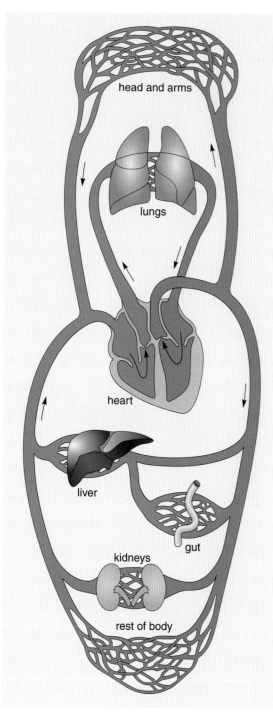

Figure 4.3 The path of blood circulation around the body. Oxygenated blood is shown in red and deoxygenated blood is shown in blue.

Another book in this series, *Trauma, Repair and Recovery* (Phillips, 2008) describes more about the structure and function of different blood vessels.

4.2 The blood circulation

Each inspiration brings air rich in oxygen into the lungs. Oxygen diffuses into the pulmonary capillaries, and enters the blood circulation carried by haemoglobin in the erythrocytes (red blood cells). The blood is pumped around the body by the action of the heart (Figure 4.3).

◆ In Figure 4.3, look at the path that the oxygenated blood takes after it leaves the heart. Can you suggest what else the blood picks up and delivers to the cells of the body?

◆ The blood also picks up nutrients from the digestion of food molecules in the gut.

The heart is composed of a series of muscles that form a double pump (Figure 4.3). The left side of the heart receives blood from the lungs that is rich in oxygen and pumps it around the rest of the body. The right side of the heart receives blood that has returned from the body tissues (and is low in oxygen and high in waste carbon dioxide from cellular respiration) and pumps it back into the lungs where exchange of gases can take place. The heart is made up of four chambers (Figure 4.4) with muscular walls. Blood enters the two *atria* (ay-tree-ah) which contract, squeezing the blood into the *ventricles* (ven-trick-ls). The two ventricles then contract very powerfully pushing the blood out forcefully around the body. There are four 'one-way' valves that allow blood to pass through only in the correct direction.

The oxygenated blood from the lungs enters the left atrium and is pumped out of the left ventricle into the system of blood vessels called **arteries** that carry it to the body tissues. The blood passes through a network of increasingly smaller blood vessels, eventually entering the tiny blood capillaries that pass close to every cell in the tissues.

◆ The tissues have a very low oxygen partial pressure (P_{O_2}) because they are using up oxygen for cellular respiration. What will happen to the oxyhaemoglobin in the blood passing through the tissues? (You might want to look back at Section 4.1.)

◆ Some of the oxyhaemoglobin will dissociate, releasing free oxygen which diffuses into the tissues.

Oxygen-depleted blood that has passed through the tissues is transported back to the heart through blood vessels called **veins**. It enters the heart at the right atrium, and is pumped out of the right ventricle via the pulmonary artery and off to the lungs where oxygen is replenished.

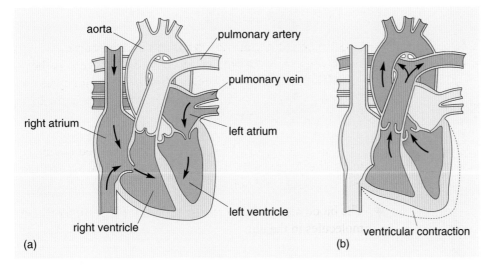

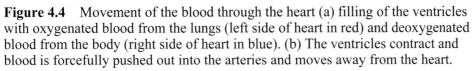

(a)   (b)

Figure 4.4   Movement of the blood through the heart (a) filling of the ventricles with oxygenated blood from the lungs (left side of heart in red) and deoxygenated blood from the body (right side of heart in blue). (b) The ventricles contract and blood is forcefully pushed out into the arteries and moves away from the heart.

4.3   Supplying sufficient oxygen to the tissues

The organs of the body require different amounts of oxygen depending on their level of activity and their requirement for energy. At rest, the body muscles or *skeletal muscles* consume about 20% of the oxygen in the blood, but this can increase to 90% during vigorous exercise when stronger and more frequent muscle contractions are required. How does the body match the requirement for oxygen with supply to the tissues? Breathing control is regulated by a complex system of sensors in the body that feed information to the respiratory centres in the brain, which in turn send out signals to the diaphragm and rib muscles to contract at an appropriate rate (Section 3.2.2). The sensors, called **chemoreceptors**, are groups of cells that convert chemical signals into action potentials that travel along nerves. Central chemoreceptors in the brain detect high blood carbon dioxide levels by monitoring the acidity of the blood (Section 4.4), while peripheral chemoreceptors in the larger blood vessels detect low blood oxygen levels (Figure 4.5 overleaf). The respiratory centres in the brain coordinate information received as action potentials from all of these sensors, and constantly adapt the rate of ventilation of the lungs. In fact an increase in carbon dioxide partial pressure (P_{CO_2}) in the blood rather than a decrease in oxygen partial pressure (P_{O_2}) is the strongest stimulus to breathe more deeply and more frequently. During rest, blood P_{CO_2} is low and so the ventilation rate is low.

◆   Why does blood P_{CO_2} increase during strenuous exercise?

◆   Exercise increases the requirement for cellular respiration to provide the necessary energy for muscle contraction. More of the products of cellular respiration (carbon dioxide and water) are therefore produced by the tissues.

The carbon dioxide diffuses into the blood stimulating an increase in ventilation rate ensuring that more oxygen is delivered to the muscles and other organs.

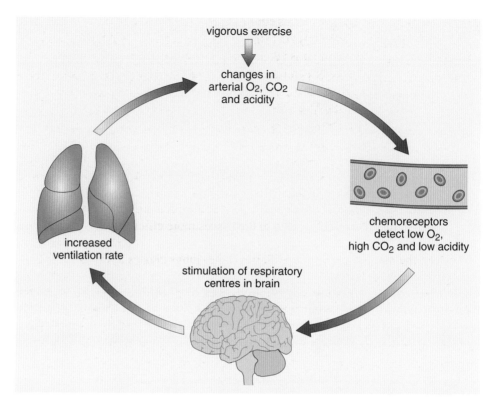

Figure 4.5 Greater exertion increases the rate of cellular respiration, increasing blood carbon dioxide levels and the demand for oxygen. Chemoreceptors in the brain and the large blood vessels detect the changes in carbon dioxide and oxygen levels in the blood and transmit action potentials along nerves to the respiratory centres in the brain. These in turn transmit an increased rate of action potentials to the muscles that drive ventilation, increasing the rate of breathing.

Epinephrine is often referred to as adrenalin.

Strenuous exercise also stimulates the adrenal (or suprarenal) glands near the kidneys to release a hormone called **epinephrine** (eppy-neff-rin) into the bloodstream. **Hormones** are molecules that are secreted into the blood somewhere in the body and are then carried to another site in the body where they bind to cells in certain organs or tissues and stimulate them to make some sort of response (Chapter 7). Epinephrine stimulates an increase in the force and rate of the heartbeat, and also causes the blood capillaries in the skeletal muscles to widen, or dilate, so that more blood flows into the muscles, helping to deliver oxygen more quickly.

◆ What would happen to the muscles during exercise if the supply of oxygen could not be increased?

◆ The muscles would not be able to generate enough energy to sustain rapid contractions for very long, and they would become fatigued.

Vignette 4.2 considers the effect of COPD on blood circulation.

Vignette 4.2   Bibi Gul's COPD causes pulmonary hypertension

Another consequence of the complex response of the body to low oxygen and high carbon dioxide levels is that Bibi Gul's body has constricted (narrowed) the blood capillaries in her lungs to slow down the flow of blood through her lungs.

◈   Can you suggest why this might help to alleviate the shortage of oxygen in her damaged lungs and help to combat her hypoxia?

◆   Slowing the flow of blood through the pulmonary capillaries gives more time for the erythrocytes to pick up oxygen molecules that do diffuse through the alveolar walls. This helps to keep the P_{O_2} of the circulating blood a little bit higher so that it delivers oxygen to the tissues more efficiently.

However, the narrowing of the capillaries in her lungs creates a resistance to the blood entering the lungs (Figure 4.3). Blood 'backs up' towards the right ventricle of the heart creating **pulmonary hypertension**, meaning very high blood pressure pressing against the walls of the pulmonary artery. High blood pressure is a sign that, somewhere in the body, the passage of blood through the circulation is impeded. The right ventricle of Bibi Gul's heart has to work much harder to push blood out against the restricted flow, and over time the right side of her heart has become stretched and enlarged (this is referred to by the Latin term *cor pulmonale* (core-pull-mon-ah-lee)) and possibly damaged. The high blood pressure can in fact back up right through the heart and affect the veins returning deoxygenated blood from the tissues to the right atrium of the heart. High pressure in these veins causes fluid from the blood to be squeezed out into the surrounding tissues. Because of this, Bibi Gul has uncomfortable swelling of her ankles, legs and feet where the blood is farthest from the heart and its movement up the legs is opposed by the effects of gravity. 'Water on the ankles' is an expression commonly used to describe this condition.

4.3.1 Oxygen and cognitive function

You are familiar now with the idea that oxygen is vital to all the organs of the body and the brain is no exception. Although the brain is only 2% of the body's total weight, it receives about 20% of the blood supply. If brain cells lose their supply of oxygen from the blood they will be irreversibly damaged within minutes. The brain constantly regulates its own blood supply, and as different parts of the brain become active their blood supply increases to replenish oxygen levels. **Cognitive functions** such as decision-making, remembering, paying attention, following a conversation, and creative thinking all suffer if blood oxygen levels are low. When oxygen levels are dangerously low it can be difficult to complete simple tasks, or even to care about doing so.

◈   Why might aircraft safety instructions stress that during an emergency you should secure your own oxygen mask in place before helping anyone else?

◆   If your own oxygen levels get too low you may behave in confused and unpredictable ways and may fail to help anyone else or even yourself.

So for people with COPD, it is not only physical activity that is compromised. Confusion and a reduced ability to solve problems in daily life may make them less able to make adjustments to their disease, and reduced memory capacity may affect lifestyle and even adherence to COPD treatment regimes such as taking drugs regularly. Vignette 4.3 explains how oxygen therapy may benefit people with COPD.

Vignette 4.3   Bibi Gul requires oxygen therapy

Bibi Gul's severe COPD is becoming quite dangerous. As the oxygen partial pressure (P_{O_2}) of her blood falls, and the carbon dioxide partial pressure (P_{CO_2}) rises, she starts to become increasingly drowsy and confused and may eventually lose consciousness as her brain shuts down. She could stop breathing altogether. The best treatment for Bibi Gul would be to breathe pure oxygen for most of the day.

◆ Why would breathing 100% oxygen rather than air help Bibi Gul?

◆ During inspiration oxygen diffuses from the alveoli into the blood capillaries until it reaches an equal pressure on both sides. Bibi Gul is struggling to draw air into her lungs because of the restricted airflow through her lungs, so breathing 100% oxygen instead of air (which is only 21% oxygen) compensates for this by raising the oxygen gas pressure inside her lungs, so that more molecules of oxygen will diffuse into her blood at each inspiration.

Unfortunately tanks of pure oxygen, although widely available in affluent countries, are only available in the health clinics of a large town hundreds of miles away from Bibi Gul's home, so she is unable to have this treatment even during an exacerbation of her COPD. Her only strategy is to keep as still as possible to reduce her requirement for oxygen. The lack of access to emergency medical treatment such as oxygen contributes to the relatively low life expectancy in countries such as Afghanistan (in 2004, average life expectancy at birth was 42 years for Afghani men and women (WHO, 2006)).

4.4   The exchange of gases between the blood and the body tissues

As oxygenated blood passes through blood capillaries in the tissues, the haemoglobin releases oxygen.

◆ What will be the consequences for Bibi Gul's tissues of the low oxygen levels in her blood?

◆ The concentration gradient between the oxygen in her blood and tissues will not be very great. Compared with a person with healthy lungs, less oxygen will diffuse into her tissues which will not be able to carry out cellular respiration efficiently.

Respiration doesn't just deliver oxygen to the tissues, it also removes the waste gas carbon dioxide that is constantly produced by cellular respiration. Carbon dioxide is a small molecule that, like oxygen, can diffuse freely through cell membranes.

◈ What do you think will happen to waste carbon dioxide that builds up in Bibi Gul's cells due to cellular respiration?

◆ When carbon dioxide inside a cell reaches a higher concentration than that outside the cell, it will leave the cell by diffusion across the cell membrane and some will enter the nearby blood capillaries.

The carbon dioxide is transported in the blood to the lungs where is can be expelled. However, the ability of Bibi Gul's lungs to exchange oxygen and carbon dioxide with the external atmosphere is reduced by her emphysema and chronic bronchitis. The level of carbon dioxide circulating in her blood will gradually build up because it is constantly produced by cellular respiration and cannot be removed as rapidly as it would be in a person with healthy lungs. In this section, we will explore how carbon dioxide is removed from the body, and why the build-up of carbon dioxide is toxic.

When carbon dioxide enters the blood from the tissues, some of it simply dissolves in the blood *plasma* (the liquid part surrounding the erythrocytes), and some binds to haemoglobin, although unlike oxygen it binds to the globin proteins, not the haem. However, most of the carbon dioxide (90%) reacts with water inside the erythrocytes to form electrically charged atoms or group of atoms called **ions** (Box 4.1 overleaf). These are negatively charged bicarbonate ions (HCO_3^-) and positively charged hydrogen ions (H^+) (Equation 4.1):

$$CO_2 + H_2O \underset{}{\overset{\text{carbonic anhydrase (enzyme)}}{\rightleftharpoons}} H^+ + HCO_3^- \qquad (4.1)$$

carbon dioxide   water   hydrogen ion   bicarbonate ion

The symbol with the two half arrows pointing in opposite directions indicates that this reaction is reversible – it can go either way: forward (carbon dioxide and water react to form bicarbonate ions and hydrogen ions), or backwards (bicarbonate ions and hydrogen ions react to form carbon dioxide and water). The molecules on each side of the equation are therefore both reactants and products. This special type of reaction is called an *equilibrium reaction* because it tends to move towards a point at which the forward reaction proceeds at the same rate as the reverse reaction, so that the amounts of reactants and products on each side will reach a stable level, and won't change. At this point, the reaction is at equilibrium. You could think of it as a see-saw equally balanced by a person sitting on each end. Things will only start to change again if the reaction is unbalanced by adding or removing some of the reactants or products.

If, for instance, there is an *increase* in the concentration of carbon dioxide, then the reaction tips *forward* producing more bicarbonate and hydrogen ions and moving it back towards equilibrium. If there is a reduction in the concentration of carbon dioxide, the reaction goes in the other direction and carbon dioxide and water are formed, again moving the reaction back towards equilibrium. Both the forward and reverse reactions take place in erythrocytes through the action of an enzyme called carbonic anhydrase. The forward reaction, which produces hydrogen ions, has an important effect on the acidity of body fluids (Box 4.1).

Box 4.1 (Explanation) Hydrogen ions and acidity

Atoms are formed from *negatively* (–) charged particles called **electrons** that move around a nucleus containing particles called neutrons that have no charge and **protons** that have *positive* (+) charge. The opposite charges exactly balance each other so that overall the atom is 'neutral'; it has no electrical charge. For example, a hydrogen atom has one positive proton balanced by one negative electron, and an oxygen atom has eight positive protons balanced by eight negative electrons. However, if an atom loses an electron, it will become positively charged overall, or if it gains an electron it will become negatively charged. Acids are substances that separate or *dissociate* in a solution, releasing a positively charged hydrogen ion (H^+) and a corresponding negatively charged ion. Equation 4.2 shows the dissociation of hydrogen chloride when it dissolves in water to form hydrochloric acid:

$$HCl(aq) = H^+(aq) + Cl^-(aq) \qquad (4.2)$$

Acidity is measured using the **pH scale** (Figure 4.6), which ranges from 0 (strongly *acidic*) to 14 (strongly *basic*). The hydrogen ion concentration in any solution determines how acidic it is. Pure water is pH 7 which is *neutral* (neither acidic nor basic). An acidic solution has a *high* concentration of hydrogen ions and a *low* pH (less than 7). With a pH of about 1.5, the gastric juice in the stomach is the most acidic substance in the human body.

At the other end of the scale are *basic* solutions (commonly called alkalis (al-kah-lies)) with a pH *greater* than 7. Bases (alkalis) dissociate releasing a negatively charged hydroxide ion (OH^-). An example is sodium hydroxide (NaOH) which dissociates into a negatively charged hydroxide ion (OH^-) and a positively charged sodium ion (Na^+) (Equation 4.3).

$$NaOH(s) = Na^+(aq) + OH^-(aq) \qquad (4.3)$$

A strongly basic solution has a high concentration of hydroxide ions and a very low concentration of hydrogen ions (Figure 4.6). Household bleach (about pH 13) is very strongly basic and is a component of many household cleaning products because it is highly caustic (corrosive, it destroys living tissue).

When acidic and basic solutions are added together they react to 'neutralise' each other. If hydrochloric acid and sodium hydroxide solutions are mixed (the two solutions represented by Equations 4.2 and 4.3), the hydrogen and hydroxide ions react together to form water, and the sodium and chloride ions remain as aqueous ions in solution. If an equal number of hydrogen and hydroxide ions are present, a neutral solution (pH 7) containing Na^+ and Cl^- ions is produced; this solution is the same as a solution of salt (NaCl) in water.

$$HCl(aq) + NaOH(aq) = Na^+(aq) + Cl^-(aq) + H_2O \qquad (4.4)$$

A hydrogen ion (which has one positive charge and no electron) is actually the same as a proton, and the two terms are often used interchangeably.

In a chemical equation, the terms in brackets show the physical states: g is gas, l is liquid s is solid, and aq indicates an aqueous solution (dissolved in water).

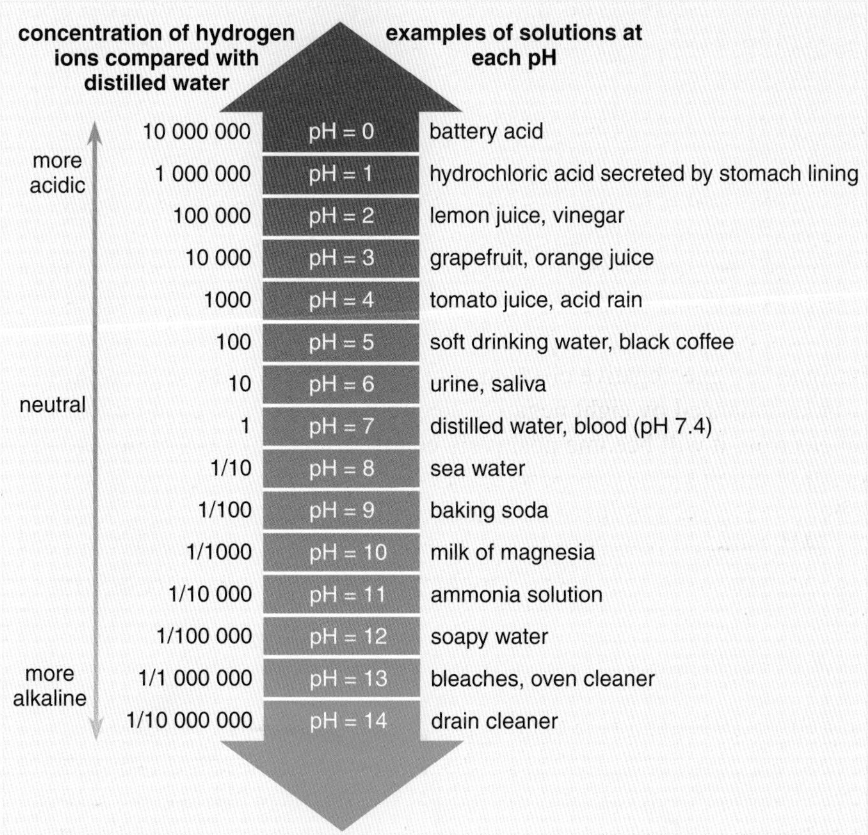

Figure 4.6 The pH of some familiar solutions marked on the pH scale. Notice that each point on the pH scale is a 10-fold change in hydrogen ion concentration. This is known as a logarithmic scale.

If carbon dioxide levels increase in the blood, the reaction shown in Equation 4.1 will produce more H^+ and HCO_3^- ions.

◆ What effect will this have on the blood pH?

◆ It will increase the hydrogen ion concentration and therefore *lower* the blood pH.

Too much acidity (low pH) is very dangerous because most of the chemical reactions that occur in the body, especially those involving enzymes, only take place in conditions of neutral pH (around pH 7). If the body's overall pH starts to drop below 6.8 (a condition known as **acidosis** (as-id-oh-sis)), many essential processes will be inhibited. The erythrocytes are resistant to their own high *internal* H^+ ion concentrations, and in fact low pH inside the erythrocytes speeds up the release of oxygen from the haemoglobin molecules packed into these cells.

◆ Why might this be beneficial in normal circumstances?

◆ The haemoglobin will release oxygen more quickly as the erythrocytes pass through the tissues where the carbon dioxide concentration is *high* and the pH of the blood becomes *low*.

When the deoxygenated blood returns to the lungs where carbon dioxide levels are low, the enzyme carbonic anhydrase converts bicarbonate and hydrogen in the blood cells back into carbon dioxide and water. The carbon dioxide diffuses out of the pulmonary capillaries into the alveoli and is expelled from the body as carbon dioxide gas in the next expiration. As well as delivering oxygen, the lungs therefore also help to maintain the body's neutral pH by eliminating carbon dioxide. In emphysema, obstruction of the lungs reduces the ability to expel the carbon dioxide by expiration. Hydrogen and bicarbonate ions can therefore build up to high levels in the blood. The kidneys can compensate to some extent by secreting hydrogen ions in the urine, but people with COPD may experience the symptoms of acidosis and this may be contributing to Bibi Gul's symptoms. In Chapter 6, you will learn about the blood tests that can be used to monitor the efficiency of lung function by measuring the levels of oxygen and carbon dioxide dissolved in the blood, and the pH of the blood.

Now try Activity 4.1.

Activity 4.1   The symptoms of COPD

Allow 30 minutes

Now would be the ideal time to carry out this activity on the DVD associated with this book. It is an interactive quiz that tests how much you have learnt about COPD symptoms. Roll the cursor over the icons representing different parts of the body to reveal self-assessment questions. Once you have attempted each question you can see our answer by clicking on the body part icon. If you are unable to study this activity now, continue with the rest of the chapter and return to it as soon as you can.

Summary of Chapter 4

4.1   Oxygen is carried by oxyhaemoglobin inside the red blood cells (erythrocytes) and released in the tissues where oxygen concentration is low.

4.2   Toxic gases, such as carbon monoxide, found in air pollution bind to haemoglobin and reduce the amount of oxyhaemoglobin in the body, contributing to respiratory problems.

4.3   Strenuous exercise increases the demand for oxygen. Chemoreceptors in the brain and the large blood vessels detect concentration changes in blood carbon dioxide and oxygen. The information is coordinated by the respiratory centres in the brain to regulate the rate of ventilation. The hormone epinephrine (adrenalin) increases blood supply to the tissues by increasing the heart rate and force.

4.4   The lung obstruction in COPD reduces the efficiency of ventilation and limits the diffusion of oxygen from the alveoli into the pulmonary capillaries. The oxygen supply to the whole body is compromised and there are multiple consequences including muscle fatigue and reduced cognitive functioning of the brain.

4.5   Hypoxia induces constriction of the lung capillaries to try to match blood flow to oxygen supply. This causes pulmonary hypertension which over time may enlarge and damage the right side of the heart, and cause swelling of the body particularly the lower legs and feet.

4.6   Most of the carbon dioxide generated by cellular respiration reacts with water in the erythrocytes, through the action of the enzyme carbonic anhydrase, to form bicarbonate ions and hydrogen ions, which are carried back to the lungs and converted back to water and carbon dioxide. The carbon dioxide diffuses into the lung alveoli and is expelled during expiration.

4.7   COPD reduces the ability to expel carbon dioxide by expiration, and hydrogen ions build up in the blood, lowering its pH and causing acidosis. Many body processes only take place at neutral pH and are inhibited by low pH.

Learning outcomes for Chapter 4

After studying this chapter and its associated activities, you should be able to:

LO 4.1   Define and use in context, or recognise definitions and applications of, each of the terms printed in **bold** in the text. (Question 4.1)

LO 4.2   Explain how oxygen is transported around the body in the blood circulation and delivered to body's cells and tissues. (Question 4.1)

LO 4.3   Demonstrate an understanding of the pH scale. (Question 4.2)

LO 4.4   Describe the mechanisms that regulate ventilation and circulation to provide sufficient oxygen to the cells and tissues. (Question 4.3)

LO 4.5   Describe the symptoms of COPD (breathlessness, hypoxia, acidosis, muscle fatigue, cognitive defects) and explain how they are linked to lung damage. (DVD Activity 4.1)

Self-assessment questions for Chapter 4

You have also had the opportunity to demonstrate LO 4.5 in the self-assessment questions associated with DVD Activity 4.1.

Question 4.1 (LOs 4.1 and 4.2)

Carbon monoxide is a common component of smoke pollution. Why does severe carbon monoxide poisoning cause unconsciousness?

Question 4.2 (LO 4.3)

Does a solution with a pH of 5.5 have a higher or a lower concentration of hydrogen ions than a solution with a pH of 7.0?

Question 4.3 (LO 4.4)

What effect does an increased level of carbon dioxide in the blood have on the rate of ventilation?

CHAPTER 5

INFLAMMATION AND LUNG DAMAGE

Observing air caught in a shaft of sunlight reveals that even relatively clean air carries many visible dust particles. However, it is particles smaller than 10 μm that cannot easily be detected by the human eye which can cause COPD. Most particles larger than 10 μm are prevented from entering the lungs by mucus and cilia in the bronchi which sweep trapped debris upwards and outwards (Section 3.2) so that it can be removed by coughing or swallowing. Only the very smallest particles (less than 1–2 μm) tend to reach the narrowest bronchioli and the alveoli (Figure 5.1). In the alveolar regions of the lungs, there are no cilia or mucus-producing cells so any particles that have escaped the filtering system will be deposited there, causing irritation to the thin walls of the alveoli where gas exchange takes place.

You may be familiar with pictures showing black deposits of tar and particles inside the lungs of lifelong cigarette smokers. This certainly looks unpleasant, but how does the accumulation of particles result in the breathing difficulties seen in COPD patients? Examination of the lungs of people with COPD, or even healthy cigarette smokers, shows that there is a permanent state of **inflammation** in the lungs. Inflammation is the first response of the body to wounds, infection or irritation, and it is characterised by redness, heat, swelling and sometimes pain in the affected area. It is an essential part of the normal process of healing and protecting wounds. However, if inflammation is sustained for long periods, it can have disastrous consequences for body tissues.

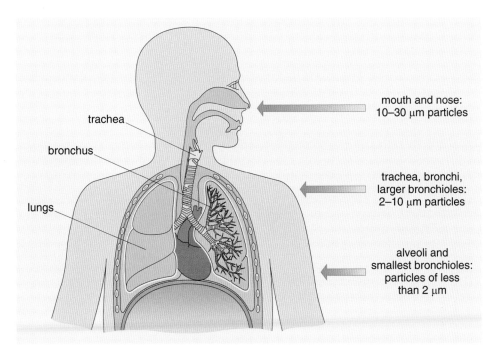

Figure 5.1   Only very small particles can reach into the smallest bronchioles and alveoli.

5.1   The immune system: the body's natural defence

Pathogens are harmful microbes such as bacteria, viruses or fungi that cause disease.

The body is constantly exposed to a whole range of potentially harmful substances including **pathogens**, as well as non-living substances such as toxins, drugs and particles. In order to protect itself, the body has a whole battery of defensive mechanisms known as the **immune system**. The first level of protection is to prevent substances and pathogens getting into the body in the first place, so there are a number of barriers to their entry including the skin, and the mucus and cilia that protect the respiratory passages. However, if a substance or pathogen breaches these barriers and enters the body tissues, there is a complex network of immune system cells and molecules which form a second line of defence. Several types of immune system cells called white cells or **leukocytes** (loo-koh-sites) patrol the body. Some are specialised cells that only recognise and kill a specific type of organism, e.g. a particular species of bacterium or virus. This type of cell can recognise a pathogen that it has encountered before, so that if the same organism infects the body a second time, it will be detected very quickly and prevented from taking hold. This is the basis of *vaccination* or immunisation against particular infectious diseases such as influenza (Section 7.2.3). Many types of leukocytes are, however, non-specific and defend the body against any type of foreign object including microbes, toxins and particles. It is this type of immune cell that, paradoxically, causes disease in COPD.

5.1.1   Inflammation protects wounds against infection

Damage to tissues creates a potential for infection, and components of the immune defence mechanisms are immediately rushed to the site of a wound.

◆ Can you recall what you observed the last time that you cut yourself accidentally?

◆ You would have felt the pain of the cut, but you would also have noticed that the whole area around the cut very quickly became inflamed (red, hot and puffed up) and remained very painful until the inflammation subsided.

The damaged cells in a wound or in lungs irritated by smoke or dust release a range of different chemicals and proteins called **inflammatory mediators** (Figure 5.2). Some of these amplify the inflammatory response by making the blood capillaries in the area *dilate* (widen), so that larger amounts of blood flow through them and the local tissue becomes red and hot. The walls of the blood capillaries become more permeable or leaky and inflammatory mediators attract leukocytes which squeeze out through the leaky capillary walls into the inflamed tissue. Blood plasma also leaks out of the capillaries and accumulates in the tissues, hence the swelling. The swelling may squeeze and stimulate the sensory endings of local *nociceptive neurons* which transmit electrical signals to the brain that are perceived as pain.

Pain and the role of nociceptive neurons is described in more detail in another book in this series (Toates, 2007).

The first leukocytes to arrive are the **phagocytes** (fag-oh-sites), literally meaning 'cells that eat'. Phagocytes attach to microbes or other small particles and completely engulf them (Figure 5.3). Once inside the phagocyte, the particle is broken down by powerful digestive enzymes. Other types of leukocytes secrete toxic chemicals that kill pathogens, or help to amplify the inflammation.

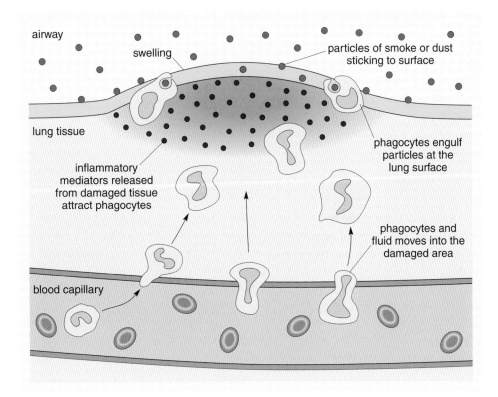

Figure 5.2 A schematic diagram of inflammation of the lung airways. Particles sticking to the surface of the airways damage cells causing the release of inflammatory mediators. These chemicals make nearby capillaries more leaky and attract circulating phagocytes into the area. Fluid leaking out of the capillaries causes swelling.

5.1.2 Inflammation can get out of control

Inflammation can occur almost anywhere in the body as a result of infection or physical damage, including in internal organs such as the heart, kidneys or lungs. It doesn't always cause pain because not all organs contain the tips of nociceptive neurons. Inflammation caused by an injury is referred to as **acute inflammation**. It occurs quickly, usually within a couple of hours, and only lasts for a few days at most. Once the damage has begun to heal, the inflammation is suppressed. However, inflammation can sometimes cause disease. Asthma is the result of an acute inflammatory response where the airways become irritated, inflamed and constricted. It can usually be successfully treated and controlled with drugs that reduce the inflammation and airway constriction (a subject we will come back to in Chapter 6). COPD is a condition where long-term or **chronic inflammation** causes irreversible damage to the lungs.

The majority of tobacco smokers have persistent inflammation of the lungs, and their lung tissues contain a large population of

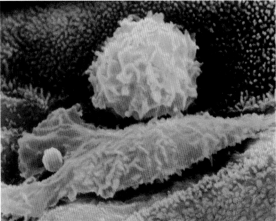

Figure 5.3 A scanning electron microscope image (magnified to about 2000 times actual size) showing two phagocytes in a human lung. The colours have been added to make objects easier to see. The phagocyte at the top is in its normal spherical shape, the one beneath it has elongated and is about to engulf the small, round particle on the left (green). (Source: Arnold Brody/Science Photo Library)

immune cells, particularly phagocytes. This seems to be a normal damage–repair response to the repeated exposure to smoke particles, and is reversible if the individual stops smoking before the process goes too far. Unfortunately, in 25% of smokers the inflammation becomes irreversible, resulting in COPD, which is sometimes diagnosed many years *after* an individual has stopped smoking. This is because the immune cells 'recruited' by the original lung damage stay in the lungs and start to damage the tissues. It is not clear why this occurs in some people and not others (Section 2.3), but we will look at why this runaway inflammation damages the lungs.

5.1.3 Chronic inflammation permanently damages the lungs

Particles and toxins sticking to the walls of the small airways and alveoli damage the cells and cause an inflammatory response. Phagocytic cells are attracted in large numbers into the lungs and release powerful protein-digesting enzymes called **proteinases** (pro-teen-ay-zes). These normally digest any microbes or particles engulfed by these cells, but if the enzymes leak into the surrounding tissues, they can begin to digest the proteins in the lung tissues as well. One of the major culprits is an enzyme called **elastase**, which phagocytes normally use to break down proteins in the cell walls of bacteria. Unfortunately elastase, as its name suggests, also breaks down a body protein called elastin.

◆ Can you recall what function elastin has? (You may want to look back at Box 3.4.)

◆ It is a component of the connective tissue fibres that give elasticity to the walls of the airways and alveoli and so aids expiration of air.

Normally, the lungs are protected from the destructive effect of elastase by the body's own natural elastase inhibitor, a protein called **alpha-1 antitrypsin** (ant-ee-tripsin) **(AAT)** which is produced by the liver and circulates through the body in the blood. Chronic inflammation, however, attracts huge numbers of phagocytes, and stimulates them to release so much elastase that eventually the AAT may be overwhelmed, and 'bystander' damage to the lung tissue occurs. The development of COPD is thought to be due to this imbalance between destructive elastase and protective AAT.

A very small number of people inherit a defective version of the gene carrying the instructions to make AAT protein (Box 5.1), and they fail to produce enough of it. They tend to develop COPD at an unusually young age, even if they have never been tobacco smokers (Needham and Stockley, 2004). These individuals however account for less than 1% of COPD cases. The great majority of people with COPD have perfectly normal AAT genes so what makes them susceptible to COPD is unclear (Section 2.3). The inflammatory response to lung damage is extremely complicated and many different types of cells and enzymes take part in ways that are not fully understood. Research into the factors that increase susceptibility to COPD may in the future help to devise strategies and therapies to combat its effects.

Box 5.1 (Explanation) An inherited defect in the gene for AAT can accelerate COPD

The manufacture of AAT by liver cells is controlled, as for all body proteins, by an inherited **gene** which carries the instructions for making the protein. Each person has two versions, called alleles (al-eels), of every gene, one inherited from each parent. Individuals who inherit *two* defective alleles of the *AAT* gene make virtually no functional AAT protein in their liver cells. The lack of AAT activity in these individuals allows the damage of tissue in the lungs by elastase to continue unopposed. This causes emphysema by the age of 30 or 40, and because of the unusually early onset, such people are sometimes misdiagnosed as having asthma not COPD. Tobacco smoking accelerates the damage.

The convention is to print gene names in italics, and the protein they encode in normal type so the *AAT* gene carries the coded instructions for making the AAT protein.

◆ What would you predict about the levels of active AAT in a person who inherits one normal and one defective *AAT* allele?

◆ They would probably have less AAT protein than is normal, but more than individuals who inherit two defective *AAT* alleles.

Individuals with at least one normal and one defective *AAT* allele don't appear have an increased risk of developing COPD if they do not smoke, presumably because they have enough AAT to cope. However, their risk of developing COPD is very high if they *do* smoke. Blood tests can find out if a person has defective *AAT* alleles, and these tests are often used during diagnosis of people who show symptoms of COPD before the age of 45 in the absence of recognised risk factors such as tobacco smoking.

5.2 The consequences of lung damage

The activity of elastase (and probably other digestive enzymes released by leukocytes) contributes to the destruction of the walls of small airways and alveoli, creating large airspaces in the lung instead of the normal fine sponge-like structure (Figure 5.4 overleaf). This reduces the lungs' elastic recoil and the small airways also lack strength and tend to collapse during expiration so that air is trapped inside the enlarged airspaces.

◆ Why would losing alveolar walls also cause problems with gas exchange between the lungs and the blood?

◆ It reduces the area for diffusion of gases, so that less oxygen gets into the blood, and less carbon dioxide leaves the blood.

Chronic inflammation causes swelling of the walls of the bronchioles as fluid floods in from the capillaries and it stimulates the secretion of large amounts of mucus, all of which contributes to obstruction of the airways, and the difficult, wheezy breathing that is experienced in chronic bronchitis. The inflammation damage eventually triggers repair processes in which special cells lay down a

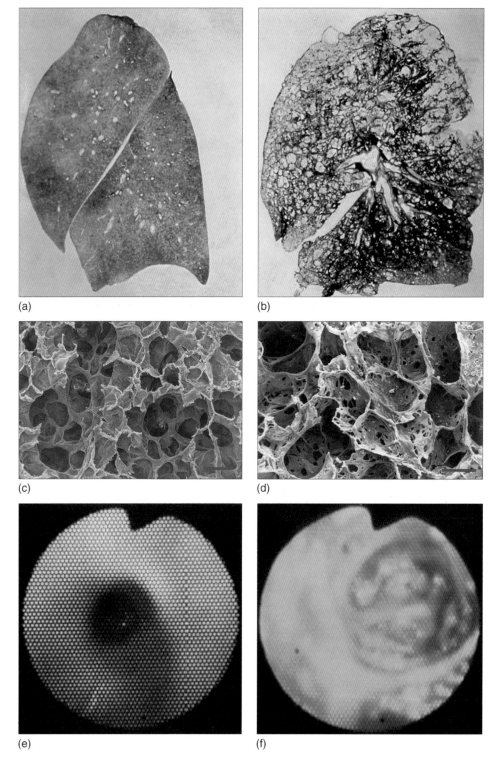

Figure 5.4 (a) A normal lung and (b) a lung from a patient with advanced emphysema (Source: Wellcome Photo Library). (c) A scanning electron microscope image (×50 magnification) showing alveoli in the lungs of a non-smoker and (d) in a person with emphysema; the loss of alveolar walls gradually enlarges the airspaces in the lungs (Source: Jeffery, 2000, Figure 8, p. 256S). (e) A view down a clear, open bronchiole of a healthy person and (f) a person with chronic bronchitis showing a folded, irregular surface obstructing a bronchiole (Source: Kikawada et al., 2000, Figures 1 and 2, p. 107)

protective layer of 'scar tissue', a type of replacement connective tissue, on the damaged surfaces. The continuous laying down of scar tissue gradually thickens the walls of the bronchioles, narrowing the airway and permanently obstructing the passage of air. Individuals with COPD may have a mixture of emphysema, and chronic bronchitis in different proportions, but the overall result is permanent obstruction of the airways, breathlessness, chronic coughing and increased susceptibility to lung infections.

◆ What effect do you expect chronic bronchitis and emphysema to have on blood oxygen and carbon dioxide levels overall.

◆ Blood oxygen levels would be lower than normal, and carbon dioxide levels would be abnormally high.

Summary of Chapter 5

5.1   Mucus and cilia in the nasal passages and larger airways trap large airborne particles and sweep them out of the respiratory system. Only very small particles (1–2 μm) accumulate in the bronchioles and alveoli where there are no cilia or mucus.

5.2   Particles and irritating gases stimulate an inflammatory response that attracts defensive immune cells, including phagocytes whose normal role is to destroy foreign organisms or particles using proteinase enzymes.

5.3   During chronic inflammation in the lungs, phagocytes may leak their proteinases into the lung tissues where they attack elastin protein in the walls of bronchioles and alveoli. The lungs consequently become floppy and less elastic. The reduction in elastic recoil makes it more difficult to expire, and the small airways tend to collapse, trapping air in the lungs (emphysema).

5.4   The inflammatory response causes swelling and thickening of the bronchioles and an increase in mucus production all of which obstruct airflow through the lungs (chronic bronchitis).

5.5   A small proportion of people with COPD have inherited defects in the gene that produces AAT, a natural inhibitor of the destructive proteinases. They develop COPD at an early age, particularly if they smoke.

5.6   The factors that determine susceptibility to COPD in the majority of people with the disease are unclear, but could involve other inherited genetic factors or environmental effects such as previous infections, allergens or diet.

Learning outcomes for Chapter 5

After studying this chapter and its associated activities, you should be able to:

LO 5.1   Define and use in context, or recognise definitions and applications of, each of the terms printed in **bold** in the text. (Questions 5.1 and 5.2)

LO 5.2   Describe what happens in inflammation and how it normally helps to protect the body against infection. (Questions 5.1 and 5.2)

LO 5.3   Discuss how irritation and inflammation of the lungs can lead to permanent lung damage and obstruction of airflow. (Question 5.2)

Self-assessment questions for Chapter 5

Question 5.1 (LOs 5.1 and 5.2)

Briefly explain why an injured tissue in the body becomes hot and swollen at the site of damage.

Question 5.2 (LOs 5.1, 5.2 and 5.3)

Where do the proteinases that are thought to damage the lungs in COPD come from? What molecule does the body produce to try and minimise tissue damage caused by these proteinases?

CHAPTER 6

DIAGNOSING COPD

Diagnosis is the art of distinguishing one disease from another, and finally identifying the disease so that appropriate steps can be taken to treat it. There are several elements in making a diagnosis. The first is to take a *medical history*, an explanation by the patient from which a doctor should be able to extract information about symptoms, previous medical problems and possibly some family history and social background – anything that may shed light on the nature of the condition. The doctor can also make a physical examination, and carry out specialised tests which may reveal *clinical signs* of which the patient may be unaware, for example high blood pressure. Think back to the description of Jenny's symptoms, then look at Table 6.1 which compares the symptoms of COPD and asthma. There isn't much to observe physically, except Jenny's breathlessness (this is called *dyspnoea* (disp-nee-a)) and her mucus-producing cough.

Table 6.1 The symptoms of COPD compared with those of asthma. (Source: adapted from Currie and Legge, 2006, Table 1, p. 1261)

Indicator	COPD	Asthma
Age	greater than 35 years	any age
Cough	persistent and produces sputum	intermittent and doesn't produce sputum
Smoker	common	possible
Breathlessness	progressive and persistent	intermittent and variable
Symptoms occur at night	uncommon until advanced disease	common
Family history of disease	uncommon unless family members also smoke	common
Allergies (eczema, hay fever)	possible	common

◆ What questions do you think Jenny's GP would have asked to make a differential diagnosis of COPD trying to rule out asthma?

◆ The GP would have found out from Jenny that her breathlessness was persistent rather than occasional or confined to night time, and that her coughing produced sputum. Equally importantly, he would have built up a picture of her circumstances, her age and her exposure to COPD risk factors, in this case her long-term cigarette smoking habit. Also, he would have noted the fact that she and her parents haven't had problems with allergies or hay-fever.

All of these observations point to the fact that Jenny's symptoms are more likely to be due to COPD than asthma. However, confirming a diagnosis of COPD isn't particularly straightforward.

6.1 Imaging COPD

Another book in this series *Screening for Breast Cancer* (Parvin, 2007) explains how X-ray images are used in breast cancer screening.

A common way of looking inside the body is X-ray imaging which is particularly useful for viewing broken bones. However, the lungs are composed mainly of air, and the soft tissue supporting the airways isn't very dense like bone so the changes in the lung tissues caused by COPD are difficult to see. X-ray images or computerised tomography (CT) scanning (a form of X-ray imaging which can build a three dimensional picture from a series of images of slices of the body) may, however, show up a blockage caused by something else such as a tumour, and in people with advanced emphysema, they may show that the lungs are abnormally enlarged, with large airspaces called *bullae* (bull-ee) bulging out from the surface of the lungs where the airway walls have been weakened (Figure 6.1). Images such as these can help surgeons decide whether lung surgery to remove damaged lung tissue may help (Chapter 7).

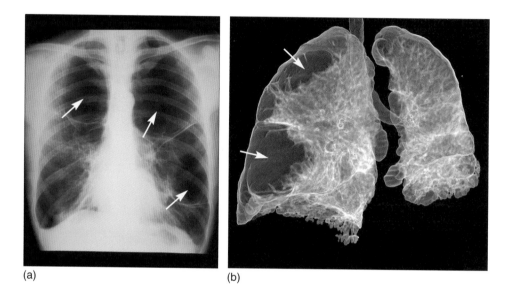

(a)
(b)

Figure 6.1   Images of the lungs of two people with severe emphysema. (a) An X-ray image of a lung with large areas of trapped air, called bullae (indicated by arrows). (Source: GJLP/CNRI/Science Photo Library). (b) A CT scan showing bullae as more transparent areas compared with the rest of the lung. (Source: Du Cane Medical Imaging Ltd/Science Photo Library)

6.2 Airflow tests to assess lung function

The alternative way of diagnosing COPD is to directly measure the efficiency of lung function. There are two aspects to this: (1) how efficiently air is inhaled and exhaled at each breath, and (2) how efficiently the oxygen is transferred from the alveoli into the blood.

The **total lung capacity (TLC)** of an adult is usually somewhere between 3 and 6 litres of air. Men usually have a larger TLC than women as they are on average physically larger. The volume of air inspired and expired with each normal breath when the body is at rest is actually a surprisingly small proportion of the total lung capacity (Figure 6.2), normally only about 0.5 litre. This fraction is called the **tidal volume (TV)**. There is a much larger reserve lung volume to allow for deeper breathing during exertion. The **vital capacity (VC)** is the maximum volume of air that can be expired starting with completely filled lungs. However, even if you expire as much air as you are able to, there is always an amount left in the lungs that you can't get out (so, in fact, the lungs can never actually be empty of air) and this is known as the **residual volume (RV)**. The total lung capacity (TLC) is therefore the sum of VC + RV (Figure 6.2).

◆ What is the TLC of the person depicted in Figure 6.2?

◆ Six litres.

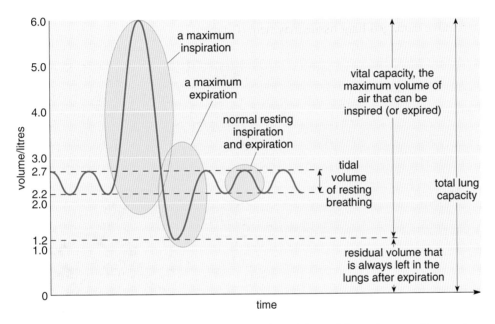

Figure 6.2 A graph representing someone breathing with a mixture of normal 'shallow' resting breaths and also consciously inspiring and expiring as much air as they can.

Vignette 6.1 explains how these volumes are measured to assess lung function.

Vignette 6.1  Jenny's lung function tests

At the local hospital's respiratory clinic Jenny is rather nervous, but the specialist respiratory nurse reassures her and explains that the test simply involves breathing into a machine, the **spirometer**, which is able to make measurements of both the volume and speed of her expirations (Figure 6.3). Jenny sits at the spirometer. She fully inflates her lungs by taking a deep breath, then seals her mouth around the tube and breathes out forcefully, keeping going until she feels that her lungs are empty. This takes several seconds. The respiratory nurse has to make sure Jenny carries out the test at least three times. The final result will only be reliable if the three tests are consistent, that is, the values they show are similar each time.

◆ Which of the above volumes (TLC, TV, VC or RV) is being measured in this test?

◆ The vital capacity (VC).

In the clinic it is referred to as the **forced vital capacity** (**FVC**) because the breath is being consciously forced out of the lungs. COPD patients take slightly longer to fully expire than someone with healthy lungs because their airways are narrower and there is less elastic recoil in the lungs to help them. The respiratory nurse can also get a quantitative measure of how efficiently Jenny can empty her lungs by measuring her **FEV_1**, or *forced expiratory volume over 1 second*. This is the amount of air that Jenny can expel during the first second of her forced expiration. A person with normal healthy lungs will be able to forcefully expel most of the air (about 80%) from their lungs in the first second. The remainder comes out more slowly. An FEV_1 of much less than that 80% will indicate that the passage of air out of Jenny's lungs is obstructed.

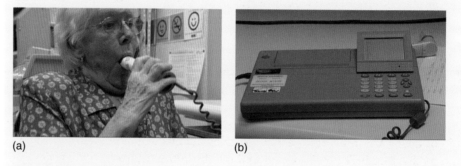

(a) (b)

Figure 6.3 (a) Taking a spirometry test. (b) A spirometer. (Source: Owen Horn/Open University)

Figure 6.4 shows the results of a spirometry test represented on a graph called a **spirogram**. The spirogram in Figure 6.4a represents the expiration of a woman (of about the same age and height as Jenny) with normal healthy lungs. The vertical axis along the side shows the total volume of air that has been expired in litres, while the horizontal axis along the bottom shows the time that has elapsed in seconds. The spirogram allows you to follow the increase over time of total volume of air expired as the person breathes out. The volume rises rapidly over the first second, then once most of the air has been expired, the curve flattens out, and the expiration is completely finished after about 6 seconds.

◆ In Figure 6.4a, what is the total volume expired in litres?

◆ The total volume expired is about 3.2 litres (read the volume from the vertical axis using the dashed line).

This value is the FVC, the total forced vital capacity.

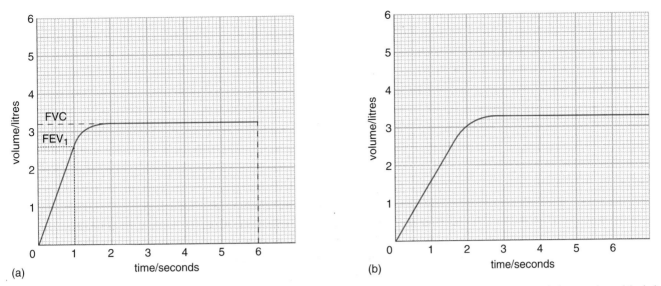

Figure 6.4   Spirograms showing the forced expirations of two women of about the same age (53 years) and height (165 cm). (a) Spirogram of a woman with normal healthy lungs. (b) Jenny's spirogram.

◆ From Figure 6.4a, what volume is exhaled in the first second?

◆ About 2.6 litres (follow the line up from the 1 second mark on the horizontal axis and read the volume from the vertical axis using the dotted line).

This value is the FEV_1 (as explained in Vignette 6.1). This person is able to expel 80% of their FVC in the first second (to calculate this work out their FEV_1/FVC ratio by dividing FEV_1 by FVC and multiply by 100% (($2.6 \div 3.2$) $\times$ 100% = 80%). Now look at Figure 6.4b which shows Jenny's test result.

◆ Use the spirogram in Figure 6.4b to identify Jenny's FVC and FEV_1 in litres.

◆ Her FVC is approximately 3.3 litres. After 1 second she had exhaled about 1.6 litres (her FEV_1 is 1.6 litres).

◆ How do Jenny's FVC and FEV_1 compare with the healthy individual represented in Figure 6.4a?

◆ Her FVC is slightly larger (3.3 litres), but her FEV_1, that is the amount of air she can force out in the first second is much lower.

So although the vital capacity of Jenny's lungs is at least as good if not better than that of the healthy woman (perhaps because she is able to hyperinflate her less elastic lungs), she is unable to force the air out at an equally high rate (it therefore takes her slightly longer to complete her expiration). This is why the condition is called an *obstructive* lung disease. Her residual volume (RV) has probably also increased (Figure 6.2), but it can't be measured by spirometry. There are other techniques that can be used to measure RV but these are outside the scope of this book.

In practice, because there isn't an ideal 'healthy person' on hand to compare with each patient, the respiratory nurse will compare Jenny's test results against a standard table (Table 6.2) showing predicted normal values that have been worked out by testing individuals with fully functional lungs. These reference values take into consideration the age, height, weight, gender and racial or ethnic background of the patient (FEV_1 and FVC, for example, are on average higher in white people compared with black or Asian people).

Table 6.2 Predictions of FEV_1 for healthy white females by age and height. (Source: based on Knudson et al., 1976)

Height/cm	145	150	155	160	165	170	175	180	185	190	195
Age/y											
10	2.06	2.20	2.33	2.47	2.60	2.74	2.87	3.01	3.14	3.28	3.41
12	2.23	2.37	2.50	2.64	2.77	2.91	3.04	3.18	3.31	3.45	3.58
14	2.40	2.54	2.67	2.81	2.94	3.08	3.21	3.35	3.48	3.62	3.75
16	2.57	2.71	2.84	2.98	3.11	3.25	3.38	3.52	3.65	3.79	3.92
18	2.74	2.88	3.01	3.15	3.28	3.42	3.55	3.69	3.82	3.96	4.09
20	2.70	2.84	2.97	3.11	3.24	3.38	3.51	3.65	3.78	3.92	4.05
25	2.60	2.73	2.87	3.00	3.14	3.27	3.41	3.54	3.68	3.81	3.95
30	2.49	2.63	2.76	2.90	3.03	3.17	3.30	3.44	3.57	3.71	3.84
40	2.28	2.42	2.55	2.69	2.82	2.96	3.09	3.23	3.36	3.50	3.63
50	2.07	2.21	2.34	2.48	2.61	2.75	2.88	3.02	3.15	3.29	3.42
60	1.86	2.00	2.13	2.27	2.40	2.54	2.67	2.81	2.94	3.08	3.21
70	1.65	1.79	1.92	2.06	2.19	2.33	2.46	2.60	2.73	2.87	3.00
80	1.44	1.58	1.71	1.85	1.98	2.12	2.25	2.39	2.52	2.66	2.79

 ◆ Jenny is 53 and her height is 165 cm. You worked out her FEV_1 and FVC in the question above. Look up the predicted normal FEV_1 value for women of Jenny's age and height using Table 6.2 to read off where the nearest age row and height column meet up. Then use a calculator to work out Jenny's FEV_1 as a percentage of the predicted 'normal' FEV_1 value that you looked up in the table. Also work out her FEV_1/FVC ratio as a percentage.

◆ Jenny has an FEV_1 of 1.6 litres and you can read off the predicted 'normal' FEV_1 value for a woman of similar age, height and ethnic group from the table as 2.61 litres. Jenny's FEV_1 is 61% of the predicted 'normal' FEV_1 (1.6 ÷ 2.61 × 100% = 61%). Jenny's FEV_1/FVC ratio is 48% ((1.6 ÷ 3.3) × 100% = 48%)

FEV_1 and the FEV_1/FVC ratio are the quantitative measurements of lung function that were used in the Platino study of COPD prevalence that you read about in Chapter 2. Table 6.3 shows the GOLD (the Global Initiative for Chronic Obstructive Lung Disease) criteria used in that study to diagnose COPD. They compare the individual's FEV_1 determined by spirometry with that predicted for someone with normal healthy lungs. They also take into account their FEV_1/FVC ratio. Remember that a person with healthy lungs should be able to expel about 80% of the air in their lungs in the first second of a forced expiration. An FEV_1/FVC ratio of less than 70% (less than 70% of the air in the lungs is expelled in the first second) indicates that lung airflow is obstructed. The GOLD criteria also take into consideration physical symptoms such as chronic coughing, shortness of breath and signs of heart failure.

In fact, the GOLD criteria stipulate that the spirometry test should be carried out after the patient has been treated with a drug called a bronchodilator that relaxes muscles in the walls of the airways (Chapter 7). This helps to ensure that airway obstruction is not the result of a reversible condition such as an asthma attack, so Jenny would have been asked to repeat the spirometry test after this treatment to make sure that her results were unchanged. You will see this being done in a respiratory clinic in DVD Activity 6.1.

Table 6.3 The GOLD classification of COPD by severity is becoming the accepted global standard for diagnosis of COPD.

Severity of COPD		Possible symptoms	Airflow limitation measured by spirometry
Stage 0	At risk	Chronic cough and sputum production.	Airflow at predicted normal level
Stage 1	Mild COPD	Mild airflow limitation and usually, but not always, chronic cough and sputum production. People with mild COPD are often unaware that they have abnormal lung function.	FEV_1‡ at least 80% of predicted normal level. FEV_1/FVC§ less than 70%. With or without symptoms.
Stage 2	Moderate COPD	Worsening airflow limitation and usually progression of symptoms such as shortness of breath on exertion.	FEV_1 less than 80% of predicted (but more than 50%). FEV_1/FVC less than 70%. With or without symptoms.
Stage 3	Severe COPD	Further worsening of airflow limitation, increased shortness of breath and repeated exacerbations* which have an impact on quality of life.	FEV_1 less than 50% of predicted (but more than 30%). FEV_1/FVC less than 70%. With or without symptoms.
Stage 4	Very severe COPD	Severe airflow limitation. Quality of life is appreciably impaired and exacerbations may be life-threatening.	FEV_1 less than 30% of predicted. FEV_1/FVC less than 70%. Also individuals with higher FEV_1 but signs of respiratory failure or right side heart failure.

* Exacerbations are periods of worsening breathing problems.
‡ FEV_1 is forced expiratory volume in 1 second measured by spirometry.
§ FVC is forced vital capacity, the total volume of a forced expiration.

◆ Compare Jenny's FEV_1 and FEV_1/FVC values with the GOLD classification of COPD severity in Table 6.3 and make an assessment of the severity of Jenny's COPD.

◆ Values of 61% of predicted 'normal' FEV_1, and an FEV_1/FVC ratio of 48% and also taking into consideration Jenny's shortness of breath on exertion, suggest she has already developed COPD that would be classified as Stage 2 or moderate.

Jenny will need to visit the respiratory clinic for regular tests to monitor her progress (Activity 6.1). We will look at what other measures she should take to manage her COPD in Chapter 7.

Activity 6.1   Testing lung function

Allow 15 minutes

Now would be an ideal time to view the video 'Testing lung function in the respiratory clinic' on the DVD associated with this book. In this video you will see a COPD patient in a respiratory clinic undergoing tests to evaluate her lung function. There are three self-assessment questions included on the DVD. These questions are repeated below for reference and you can find comments on them at the back of this book.

1   Can you suggest a reason for the angled shape of the downward slope of the COPD patients' exhalation?

2   Does the bronchodilator appear to have much effect in this case?

3   What happens to the carbon monoxide that enters the lungs?

You will find it difficult to carry on with this chapter before you have completed this activity, but if you are unable to study it now, continue with the rest of the chapter and return to it as soon as you can.

6.3   Measuring the transfer of gases between the lungs and the blood

In Activity 6.1 you saw a patient taking a gas diffusion or **gas transfer test** that measured the efficiency of the second stage of respiration; that is, how well gas passes from her lung alveoli into her blood. She inhaled air containing a known small and safe amount of carbon monoxide, some of which diffuses into the blood and binds tightly to haemoglobin molecules. She then exhaled into a machine that measured the carbon monoxide remaining in the air that she exhaled (Figure 6.5).

◆ Jenny has emphysema – so will there be more or less carbon monoxide left in the air she exhales at the end of a gas transfer test, compared with someone with healthy lungs?

◆ In emphysema, many of the alveolar walls have been destroyed, so Jenny's lungs effectively have a lower surface area, *reducing* her ability to transfer gases from her lungs into her blood. Therefore there will be *more* carbon monoxide remaining in the air that she exhales, compared with a person with healthy lungs taking the test.

6.3.1 Measuring the levels of oxygen and carbon dioxide in the blood

An **arterial blood gas test (ABG test)** directly measures the partial pressure of oxygen and carbon dioxide in the blood. It involves taking a sample of arterial blood from the wrist or elbow.

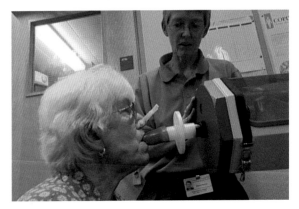

Figure 6.5 A gas transfer test to measure the efficiency of transfer of gases from the lungs to the blood. (Source: Owen Horn/Open University)

◆ Can you suggest why blood is taken from arteries carrying blood from the heart to the tissues rather than from veins carrying blood from the tissues to the heart?

◆ To get an accurate idea of how much oxygen has entered the blood, the test must be made on oxygenated arterial blood that has just left the heart after passing through the lungs. Blood in the veins has passed through the tissues and given up most of its oxygen.

As COPD progresses, reduction in the exchange of gases between the alveoli and the blood capillaries will mean that an arterial blood gas test will show an abnormally low P_{O_2} (hypoxia) and high P_{CO_2} (hypercapnia (hy-per-cap-nee-ah)). The ABG test also measures the pH (the acidity) of the blood which indicates whether a build-up of carbon dioxide in the blood is causing acidosis (Section 4.4). The ABG test is used in cases of advanced emphysema to determine whether long-term oxygen therapy is needed (Section 7.2.5). In some patients in the earlier stages of emphysema, hyperventilation may help to keep the blood gas levels relatively normal, even though the patient constantly feels breathless.

Blood cell counts may also show increased numbers of erythrocytes in people with COPD. This is an adaptation that the body makes when it is starved of oxygen. Endurance athletes often train at high altitudes where the oxygen content of air is much lower, in order to force their bodies to produce more erythrocytes to compensate. The athletes are hoping that this will improve the delivery of oxygen and the function of their muscles when they compete at lower altitudes.

Not all arteries carry oxygenated blood: the pulmonary artery carries deoxygenated blood from the heart to the lungs and the pulmonary vein carries oxygenated blood from the lungs to the heart (Figure 4.4).

6.3.2 Pulse oximetry

Having arteries punctured to take a blood sample is a painful procedure, so instead of regular ABG tests patients can be monitored, often at home, using a *non-invasive* technique called **pulse oximetry**. A pulse oximeter is a machine consisting of a probe that is attached to the patient's finger or ear lobe and linked to a computer that monitors the percentage of haemoglobin that is saturated with oxygen (i.e. how much of it is oxyhaemoglobin), together with their heart rate. The probe emits light of two wavelengths that can penetrate the skin. The light is partly absorbed by haemoglobin in amounts that differ depending on whether the haemoglobin is saturated with oxygen (bright red) or not (dark red). By calculating the amount of light absorbed, the computer can calculate the proportion of haemoglobin that is oxygenated.

Summary of Chapter 6

6.1   The diagnosis of COPD combines lung function testing and consideration of the individual's history, including age and tobacco smoking or other exposure to smoke, dust or gases.

6.2   Spirometry testing is an easy and efficient method of measuring the airflow through the lungs to identify airway obstruction. Taking the test after treatment with a bronchodilator can help to distinguish between COPD and reversible lung conditions such as asthma.

6.3   The second stage of respiration, the transfer of gases between the alveoli and the blood can be measured using a gas transfer test, as well as direct measurements of blood oxygen and carbon dioxide partial pressure and pH.

Learning outcomes for Chapter 6

After studying this chapter and its associated activities, you should be able to:

LO 6.1   Define and use in context, or recognise definitions and applications of, each of the terms printed in **bold** in the text. (Questions 6.1 and 6.3)

LO 6.2   Discuss how COPD is defined and diagnosed. (Question 6.2)

LO 6.3   Explain the principles of the tests that are used to determine the severity of COPD. (Questions 6.1, 6.3 and DVD Activity 6.1)

LO 6.4   Interpret the data from lung function tests to draw conclusions about respiratory function. (Question 6.3 and DVD Activity 6.1)

Self-assessment questions for Chapter 6

You have also had the opportunity to demonstrate LOs 6.3 and 6.4 in the self-assessment questions associated with Activity 6.1.

Question 6.1 (LOs 6.1 and 6.3)

Which of the following lung volumes could *not* be measured or calculated using a spirometry test? Explain your answer. You may want to look at Figure 6.2.

(a) Tidal volume; (b) total lung capacity; (c) residual volume; (d) vital capacity.

Question 6.2 (LO 6.2)

Explain what it means to take a medical history of a patient, and why taking a history is particularly important when making a diagnosis of COPD.

Question 6.3 (LOs 6.1, 6.3 and 6.4)

Would you expect FEV_1 to increase or decrease (compared with the predicted FEV_1 of a person with healthy lungs) during (a) an asthma attack, and (b) as a result of COPD? Explain why in each case.

CHAPTER 7

MANAGING COPD

7.1 How COPD affects patients' lives

It can be difficult to assess how much a condition like COPD affects quality of life for different people. Figures 7.1–7.3 show data from a questionnaire survey of 573 people (whose ages ranged from 45 to over 75 years) with COPD in the USA (Schulman, Ronca and Bucuvalas Inc., 2001). Of course the results of this one study may not reflect the experiences of people living in other countries.

7.1.1 The social and economic impact of COPD

Nearly a quarter (23%) of the people surveyed felt that their COPD had made them an invalid (Figure 7.1) and even more were worried about lack of control over their breathing, exacerbations, panic attacks and the embarrassment of coughing in public. 48% found it difficult to make future plans and 66% expected their condition to get worse.

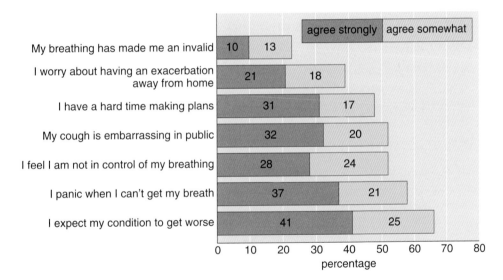

Figure 7.1 The impact of COPD on 573 people in the USA from a survey published in 2001. The question here was, 'Would you agree strongly, agree somewhat, disagree somewhat or disagree strongly with each of the following statements…' (Source: Schulman, Ronca and Bucuvalas Inc., 2001, Figure 17)

Most people in the survey said that their COPD limited what they could do in relation to many aspects of their lives (Figure 7.2 overleaf). Breathlessness prompts many people to abandon their physical and social activities which further reduces their tolerance to exercise, their mobility and their independence and can lead to a diminished role within society and the family, and the loss of intimacy in personal relationships. Some people become housebound and heavily reliant on family or welfare support for physical care. In Activity 7.1 you will compare the concerns of people in the USA survey with those of the people in the 'Living with COPD' video that you viewed in Chapter 1.

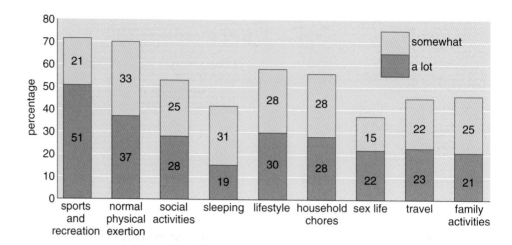

Figure 7.2 COPD limits what people can do. The survey question here was, 'How much do you feel your respiratory condition limits what you can do in each of the following areas?' (Source: Schulman, Ronca and Bucuvalas Inc., 2001, Figure 17)

Activity 7.1   What effects of COPD are important to individuals?

Allow 10 minutes

Look back at your notes on Activity 1.1 'Living with COPD'. From the comments of the people in the Breazers group featured in the video, identify which of their concerns correspond with those identified in the USA survey. Comments on this activity are included at the end of this book.

Half of the participants in the USA survey also reported that their condition either limited their ability to work or prevented them from working (Figure 7.3). In fact, this may be an underestimate of the effects on working individuals, because over half of the participants in this survey were already retired. Loss of working days has a major impact on individuals in financial terms. In developing countries, particularly poor rural communities where there is no emergency medical or welfare support, this can lead to severe financial hardship.

◆ What costs to *societies* are likely to result from a growing proportion of the population with COPD?

◆ There are the direct costs of providing healthcare and support, but also the *indirect* costs of a cumulative loss of productivity due to absence from work, or premature retirement of both people with COPD and family members who care for them.

In 2005 it was estimated that one in eight of all medical admissions to UK hospitals (approximately 100 000 admissions a year, with an average length of stay of 10 days) are a result of exacerbations of COPD (National Institute for Health and Clinical Excellence, UK).

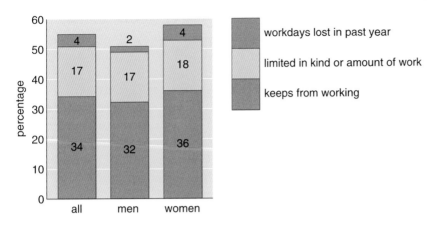

Figure 7.3 COPD limits the ability to work. The survey questions here were, 'Does your COPD keep you from working?', 'Are you limited in the kind or amount of work you can do?' and 'Have you missed work in the past 12 months due to your COPD?' (Source: Schulman, Ronca and Bucuvalas Inc., 2001, Figure 17)

7.1.2 Depression and anxiety in COPD

The combination of debilitating symptoms and poor future outlook makes people with COPD susceptible to depression, anxiety and distress. Research studies suggest that 40–60% of those with COPD experience clinically significant depression and anxiety (van Ede et al., 1999; Dowson et al., 2001) and less extreme levels of distress are even more widespread. COPD progressively reduces competence at physical, social and mental activities. Simple tasks or activities around the home may become laboured and stressful, causing frustration and embarrassment. Because the disease is often associated with past or current smoking or occupations, it can also bring with it a sense that the situation was avoidable, with associated feelings of self-blame. Often mental difficulties are not addressed because health professionals concentrate on treating the physical symptoms of COPD.

Take a moment to think about what the enjoyable activities in your everyday life are and make a mental list. How many items on your list involve increased activity or getting out of the home? Most people throughout the world enjoy some solitary sedentary entertainments such as reading or watching television, but research suggests that the types of activity that most reliably raise our sense of wellbeing and sustained pleasure frequently involve mental effort, physical activity and social interaction. Physical exercise is well known to improve mood, at least among those who lead relatively sedentary lives (Berger and Motl, 2000) as is spending time with friends, the sense of triumph at surmounting a mental or physical challenge or participating in novel stimulating activities (Lyubomirsky et al., 2005).

◆ Can you identify any reasons why even a chat with friends may be difficult for people with COPD?

◆ Talking requires breathing control, so even having a conversation can be exhausting.

Not only is depression damaging to quality of life, it might also jeopardise the ability to obtain or use treatments and may increase the risk of a poor outcome. Depression and anxiety can be alleviated by both drug and non-drug interventions. Although exercise is difficult for those with COPD, carefully chosen activities can successfully enhance mood and wellbeing, as well as improving tolerance of exercise (Section 7.2.4). Tackling depression may require an individual to learn new coping strategies that allow them to break out of a vicious cycle of low motivation, low levels of activity and reduced interest in life, leading to further reduction of activities that could provide a sense of achievement or improve physical health.

7.1.3 Panic attacks

If you have tried to hold your breath for a long time you will have noticed how dominant the urge to breathe becomes. A so-called *suffocation alarm* is activated by changes in oxygen and carbon dioxide partial pressures in the blood, alerting the body by an increase in anxiety accompanied by the release of stress hormones such as epinephrine (Section 4.3). The release of epinephrine increases ventilation rate and heart rate. Changes in blood flow around the body lead to symptoms such as butterflies in the stomach. These are normal reactions to stress, but in some people they appear to be interpreted as having life-threatening consequences and may escalate into a panic attack, releasing further epinephrine and heightening the symptoms. Whereas breathing is normally an unconscious process, the suffocation alarm usually brings it to full consciousness (Vignette 7.1).

Vignette 7.1   Jenny suffers from panic attacks

On a couple of occasions when she has had a chest infection or over-exerted herself, Jenny has experienced severe problems with breathing and has had a panic attack. She is suddenly filled with an overwhelming fear that she is going to suffocate. Her rate of ventilation increases dramatically, her heart races, she trembles and has 'butterflies' in her stomach. She feels that she has to physically force the air in and out of her lungs. The panic attack itself increases her breathing difficulties and her family has to try to calm her down before her breathing improves again.

◆ Why might some COPD patients experience panic attacks when they attempt to become more active?

◆ Changes in blood gases trigger hyperventilation, and the increased effort of breathing can itself trigger anxiety and the release of epinephrine.

People with breathing difficulties often develop an oversensitive suffocation alarm, may constantly feel anxious and are prone to panic attacks. Through fear of the possible consequences, they may avoid activity. As a result their lives can become increasingly restricted and centred on resting quietly at home, greatly reducing opportunities to socialise and pursue outside interests.

7.2 Treatments for COPD

Although the damage to the lungs in COPD cannot be reversed, there are a range of treatments and interventions available in most developed countries. These have the aims of:

- preventing disease progression
- reducing symptoms
- reducing mortality rates
- preventing exacerbations
- improving exercise tolerance
- improving the health-related quality of life.

Preventing progression of the disease and reducing mortality is obviously important, but as you have seen, people with COPD are often most concerned about reducing the frequency of exacerbations, and coping with the breathlessness, muscle tiredness and coughing that threaten to restrict their lifestyle. Table 7.1 outlines possible options for achieving these aims which we will explore in this chapter.

Table 7.1 Currently available treatments and interventions for COPD.

Disease progression	Breathlessness and exercise limitation	Frequency of exacerbations	Chronic sputum-producing cough	Respiratory failure or heart failure	Maintenance of normal body weight	Anxiety and depression
Remove source of particles. Advice and nicotine supplements to aid smoking cessation.	Drugs to reduce inflammation and open the airways. Exercise training to improve exercise tolerance. Surgery to remove damaged lung tissue, or a lung transplant.	Antibiotics to treat bacterial respiratory infections. Vaccination against respiratory infections (e.g. pneumonia and influenza).	Training in techniques for productive coughing. Drugs to loosen mucus.	Oxygen therapy. Artificial ventilation to assist breathing.	Diet and exercise advice. Nutritional supplements.	Anti-depressant drugs. Counselling and advice.

◆ From the information you have read about Jenny and Bibi Gul, can you identify which of the interventions in Table 7.1 might be (a) appropriate and (b) accessible to each of them?

◆ Jenny would have access to most of the available treatments and advice about the best way to manage her condition. Her doctor could recommend strategies for stopping smoking, offer her an inhaler containing drugs that reduce inflammation and open her airways, and vaccinate her against influenza and pneumonia to reduce the chances of lung infections. Bibi Gul's condition is probably more severe than Jenny's; however, she is unlikely to have regular access to medical attention, and may not even have been diagnosed with COPD. The solution would be for her to live in a pollution-free home and have access to regular oxygen treatment, vaccinations and inhaled drug therapy, but unless there is a health clinic or hospital of a nearby town with an interest in respiratory treatment, she is unlikely to have access to any of the interventions, even in emergencies.

Bibi Gul did have a short course of anti-inflammatory drugs and antibiotics (Section 7.2.4) when she last had an exacerbation of her COPD, but the doctor who occasionally visits the area cannot provide regular courses of treatments such as drug inhalers or vaccination because they are too expensive and difficult to distribute in the remote region where she lives. COPD remains a neglected disease in many developing countries where options may be limited to reducing exposure to smoke or dust.

7.2.1 Prevention

Reducing exposure to tobacco smoke, occupational dusts and chemicals, and indoor smoke pollution slows the rate of deterioration in lung function. This has been seen most clearly from studies on tobacco smoking cessation.

◆ In Figure 7.4, what happens to susceptible individuals who stop smoking compared with those who continue to smoke?

◆ Their *rate* of FEV_1 decline is lower; that is, they lose less lung function over time. However, the decline is not reversed – they don't get any better.

You will notice that even non-smokers gradually lose lung function after age 30, but the rate of loss is much lower than it is for smokers (Fletcher and Peto, 1977). With increasing age, connective tissue proteins such as elastin are gradually lost from body tissues, which become stiffer and less elastic – a similar process leads to wrinkling of the skin. Smoking cessation is the only intervention that has been clearly demonstrated to reduce COPD progression and prolong the life of people with COPD (Anthonisen et al., 2002).

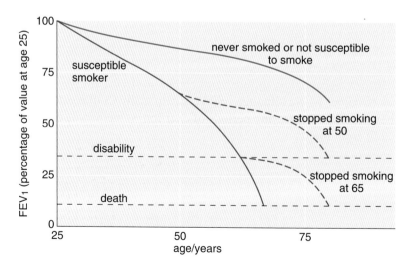

Figure 7.4 The rate of decline of lung function (current FEV_1 as a percentage of FEV_1 at age 25) in smokers who are susceptible to lung damage versus non-smokers or smokers who have a low susceptibility to lung damage.

◆ In Figure 7.4, on average how much does lifespan increase for susceptible smokers who stop smoking at age 65 compared with those who continue to smoke?

◆ It increases by approximately 15 years (although there may already be considerable disability by this stage).

7.2.2 Inhaled therapy to improve airflow

People with COPD are often prescribed inhaled drugs to relieve their symptoms. These work by mimicking the effect of hormones.

◆ What are hormones? (You may want to look back at Section 4.3.)

◆ Hormones are molecules that are secreted into the blood at one site in the body and carried in the blood to another site where they bind to cells in target tissues and stimulate them to make some sort of response.

Hormones work rather like a key in a lock. They each have a very specific shape that only fits into an appropriate type of molecule called a **receptor** on target cells. The stress hormone epinephrine prepares the body to react to threatening, exciting or stressful events by increasing ventilation rate and heart rate and changing the blood flow around the body (Section 4.3). Among its many effects are *dilation* or widening of the blood vessels supplying blood to the leg muscles (which aids a rapid escape from danger if necessary) and relaxation of the bands of muscles in the walls of the airways.

◆ What effect do you think that relaxing tight bands of muscle will have on the airways?

◆ It would dilate or widen the airways, allowing easier passage of air.

Drugs are available that have a very similar 'shape' to adrenaline, and can bind to its receptor and trigger the same response in cells – including dilation of the airways. These drugs help to relieve constriction of the bronchioles during asthma attacks, so they are called **bronchodilators** (brong-koh-dye-lay-ters) or 'relievers'. Unfortunately the bronchioles of COPD patients are often narrowed because their walls are thickened by inflammation and scar tissue, and are filled with mucus (Chapter 5). So although relievers help many COPD patients, particularly if they are taken before any periods of exertion, some people don't derive much benefit from them.

A second class of drugs (called corticosteroids) are used to treat COPD because they mimic the effects of another natural hormone called *cortisol* (cor-tee-zol) which suppresses the activity of the immune system.

◆ Why might this be helpful in reducing the symptoms of COPD?

◆ It would help to reduce inflammation in the lungs.

These **anti-inflammatories** or 'preventers' don't work quickly like bronchodilators, but taken regularly their effects are long-lived. However, currently available anti-inflammatory drugs aren't very effective at suppressing inflammation in the lungs of many COPD patients and more effective versions are being sought.

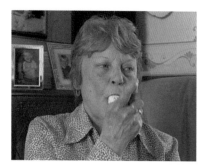

Figure 7.5   Using an inhaler. (Source: Owen Horn/Open University)

Inhalers, which squirt a fine spray of drugs (usually a combination of a bronchodilator and an anti-inflammatory) directly into the airways (Figure 7.5), are useful to many people with COPD for opening the larger airways both to improve the flow of air, and to allow sputum to be coughed out more easily. Although these drugs can help relieve symptoms and reduce the number of exacerbations, there is no evidence that they can slow the rate of progressive decline in airflow of people with COPD. In common with most drugs, they also have various **side-effects** (undesired effects), so their use has to be monitored carefully. One problem of using cortisol-like preventer drugs for long periods is that they may cause *osteoporosis* (oss-tee-oh-pore-oh-sis) a disease in which bones become fragile and more likely to break. People with COPD are usually in the older age groups who are already susceptible to osteoporosis, and their reduced mobility may also prevent them from getting the type of exercise that helps strengthen bone.

7.2.3 Clearing sputum and preventing respiratory infection

Coughing up sputum is a particularly uncomfortable and often embarrassing symptom of COPD. Preventer and reliever drugs can help to clear mucus by opening the airways. Drugs that reduce the viscosity or stickiness of the mucus can also help, as can drinking plenty of fluids and keeping the environment humid. Patients can also be taught techniques that help them to cough 'productively' such as rhythmic breathing or tapping the chest.

Mucus trapped in the lungs encourages the growth of microbes, so people with COPD are particularly vulnerable to lung infections such as influenza, or pneumonia. Pneumonia can be caused by several types of microbes including viruses and bacteria and induces such severe inflammation of the lungs that they fill up with fluid, worsening respiratory problems. Common symptoms include fever, coughing and chest pain. Recurrent or severe respiratory infections need hospital treatment, and are one of the most common causes of exacerbation and death from respiratory failure in COPD patients. Bacterial infections (but not virus infections) can be treated with antibiotics (Ram et al., 2006), although some strains of the bacteria (*Streptococcus pneumoniae*) that cause the most common form of bacterial pneumonia are becoming *resistant* to antibiotics such as penicillin. The most efficient way to tackle respiratory infections is to try to prevent them by vaccination of vulnerable members of the population, including those with COPD, against the influenza virus and the pneumococcus bacterium.

Antibiotic resistance is discussed in another book in this series (Halliday and Davey, 2007).

7.2.4 Pulmonary rehabilitation

Drugs have limited success at controlling breathlessness in COPD, so there is now increasing interest in using other strategies. **Pulmonary rehabilitation** is a multidisciplinary approach to managing COPD that aims to break the cycle of worsening breathlessness, reduced physical activity and muscle de-conditioning (Celli, 2006). It helps patients to reduce their breathlessness, improve their exercise capacity, gain a sense of control over their condition and stay physically and socially independent as long as possible (Lacasse et al., 2006) (Vignette 7.2).

Vignette 7.2 Improving Jenny's fitness and exercise tolerance

Jenny is referred for pulmonary rehabilitation, a series of weekly sessions held in a local health centre where she meets with about 20 other COPD patients. When Jenny first arrives she carries out an endurance test (a *shuttle walk test*, up and down a 10-metre course) to determine how far she can walk without becoming breathless. She is then given her own programme of gentle exercises that are designed to induce mild breathlessness and gradually improve her exercise tolerance (Figure 7.6). These are increased over time and she records her own performance and rate of improvement. The exercise therapist also encourages her to carry on with the exercises at home, and to keep up other activities such as walking. There is a respiratory nurse at the sessions who has taught Jenny to use her drug inhaler correctly, and has trained her to breathe through 'pursed-lips' when she feels particularly breathless – this reduces collapsing of the airways on expiration. There are also talks or slide shows about subjects such as diet. Some of the COPD patients at the sessions are overweight because of their lack of exercise, others are underweight because they expend a lot of their energy on breathing, and severe breathlessness may make eating difficult. Other members of the group are able to get advice about housing and disability support.

Jenny was rather reluctant to start with, and anxious that the exercise would make her condition worse, but she soon found that she enjoyed the sessions and that the health workers and the other participants were very supportive. She began to feel more in control of her COPD and once she began to learn to recognise the symptoms of an exacerbation coming on she was able to take steps to rest and relax and felt much less panicky. At the end of the 10-week course she re-took the endurance test and was very pleased with her improvement. She intends to keep to her exercise regime at home. Now try Activity 7.2 overleaf.

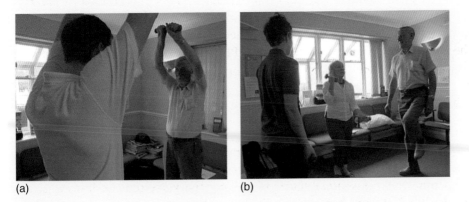

(a)   (b)

Figure 7.6 Pulmonary rehabilitation improves exercise tolerance.

Activity 7.2 Pulmonary rehabilitation

Allow 15 minutes

Now would be the ideal time to view the video entitled 'Pulmonary rehabilitation' on the DVD associated with this book. It was made with the help of the staff and participants taking part in a pulmonary rehabilitation session in Sheffield. Although pulmonary rehabilitation sessions don't appear to reduce disease progression, or increase long-term survival, they are proving very successful in improving quality of life and helping people with COPD to stay independent, especially if participants can be followed up long-term to encourage them not to revert to a sedentary lifestyle. An increase in general fitness certainly helps improve tolerance of exercise, but can you identify any other benefits of attending these exercise sessions? Write down your suggestions before reading our comment on this activity at the end of this book.

7.2.5 Treatment in advanced COPD

Patients with advanced COPD may need to spend long periods breathing pure oxygen to treat severe hypoxia and increase their chances of survival (Currie and Douglas, 2006; Ambrosino and Simonds, 2007). Oxygen gas is administered from a storage cylinder via a cannula (tube) into the nose.

◆ What test could be used to determine whether a patient has hypoxia?

◆ An arterial blood gas (ABG) test measures the levels of oxygen in arterial blood (Section 6.3.2).

Usually a patient who has an arterial blood P_{O_2} of 55 mmHg or less would be recommended to inhale oxygen for at least 15 hours a day. In many developed countries, patients can have cylinders of oxygen, or oxygen concentrators (which remove nitrogen from the air, producing oxygen-rich air) supplied to their home. Although this is a life-saving treatment, it restricts mobility. Small portable cylinders are becoming more widely available providing a couple of hours supply and allow users much more mobility (Figure 7.7). This technology is not

Figure 7.7 Portable oxygen cylinders are widely available only in some countries. (Source: Owen Horn/Open University)

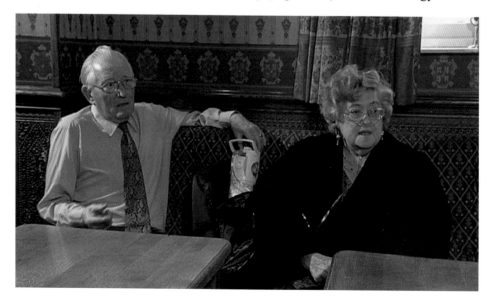

available to everyone who needs it, even in the wealthiest countries, and is out of reach of most people in other parts of the world.

Active help with breathing can also be given in hospital during exacerbations of COPD by non-invasive ventilation (NIV). This uses a device that delivers air at positive pressure (that is, higher than the normal atmospheric pressure) through a tight-fitting face mask, literally pushing air into the lungs so that the work required to breathe is decreased.

Occasionally, extremely ill patients will be given lung volume reduction surgery to remove parts of the lung that are damaged by emphysema and are full of large airspaces that trap stale air. The lung has to be stapled shut to make it airtight again. Lung volume reduction surgery can give the remaining less damaged parts of the lungs more room to inflate and recoil, improving breathing and reducing hyperventilation. Lung transplants are also possible if suitable donor organs can be identified. Again, these treatments are only available to a small proportion of those who need them. In the final chapter, we will come back to the hopes for future improvements in prevention and treatment.

Summary of Chapter 7

7.1 COPD imposes a burden of physical, emotional, social and financial stress on individuals. It also has large financial and social costs for societies.

7.2 COPD cannot be cured, but treatment aims to reduce symptoms, reduce mortality, prevent exacerbations, prevent disease progression, and improve quality of life.

7.3 Preventing further exposure to damaging particles, particularly tobacco smoking, is the only intervention that has been proven to reduce disease progression.

7.4 Several treatments are available to relieve symptoms, including inhaled drug therapy and prevention of infection using antibiotics and vaccinations.

7.5 The psychological effects of COPD can increase the debilitating physical effects by preventing people from remaining active.

7.6 Exercise rehabilitation aims to improve exercise tolerance and break the cycle of worsening breathlessness, reduced physical activity and muscle de-conditioning. It helps people to remain independent and take charge of their own health.

Learning outcomes for Chapter 7

After studying this chapter and its associated activities, you should be able to:

LO 7.1 Define and use in context, or recognise definitions and applications of, each of the terms printed in **bold** in the text. (Question 7.1)

LO 7.2 Discuss the impact of COPD on the lives of individuals. (Question 7.2 and Activity 7.1)

LO 7.3 Discuss how anxiety and depression contributes to the impact of COPD. (Question 7.2)

LO 7.4 Explain the rationale for current treatments and strategies that relieve the symptoms of COPD. (Question 7.1 and DVD Activity 7.2)

Self-assessment questions for Chapter 7

You have also had the opportunity to demonstrate LOs 7.2 and 7.4 in the self-assessment questions associated with Activity 7.1 and DVD Activity 7.2.

Question 7.1 (LOs 7.1 and 7.4)

Describe two of the benefits that COPD may derive from 'reliever'-type drugs. Why are these drugs ineffective for some people with COPD?

Question 7.2 (LOs 7.2 and 7.3)

Identify two reasons why COPD might increase social isolation.

CHAPTER 8

RECOGNISING A FORGOTTEN KILLER

A survey of 1200 UK women made by the British Lung Foundation in 2005 showed that only 1% ranked COPD as their major health concern (only 15% even included COPD in their top five). In contrast, 39% regarded breast cancer as their major health concern. In fact, the numbers of female fatalities from breast cancer and COPD in the UK are similar. Why does COPD have such low prominence in the public perception of health risks compared with other diseases such as cancer? The excerpts from two newspaper articles shown in Figure 8.1 describe some experiences of people with breast cancer or COPD.

◆ What differences can you identify in the words and attitudes included in the two reports in Figure 8.1?

◆ You probably identified some of the following words in the excerpt about cancer: fighting, campaigning, fund-raising, winning, wonder drugs, and also the individual's right to demand treatment. In contrast to this combative attitude, the report about COPD features lack of sympathy, infirmity, disability, loneliness, self-blame for smoking and an acceptance that minimal support from health services can make self-help the only option.

This week brave Emma Kearns, 28 became the latest to win her battle for treatment. Emma, a civil servant from Sutton, Surrey, starts on Herceptin next week. She says: 'I'm proof that you can fight and get the best treatment'. Cancer survivor Dorothy Griffiths, 58, was one of the first to fight for the wonder drug – after being told in 2001 her cancer was so advanced she would be dead within months. After hearing about Herceptin, the ex-NHS manager from Stoke-on-Trent started a fight for her life. She's still fighting, co-ordinating the campaign for early treatment. She says: 'Without Herceptin, I would have been six feet under long ago'. Her tips for a winning campaign are: 'Learn as much about the issue as you can, find out how the system works, get the public onside and NEVER give up. The doctors told me I would be dead within six to eight months – but I'm still here and have seen my two grandchildren born and my step-grandchildren grow up'.

Extract from an article in the *Sun* newspaper, 'Patient power – what to do if you're in a row with the NHS', 3 November 2005

A group of lung disease sufferers from Gloucester are getting together to breathe easy. With help from the British Lung Foundation, the group has formed a new support club for anyone living with or affected by a lung condition. Chairwoman Rose Durrans, who suffers from emphysema, said: 'We decided to set up the group as there is nothing like this for people in our condition in the area'. A lot of people don't realise what it's like to live with an illness like this and it can be a very lonely experience'. Breathe Easy Gloucester will offer support, advice and information on all aspects of lung disease as well as social events and the chance just to get together and talk in a relaxed and friendly place. Group secretary Dave Ward, 62, who has chronic obstructive pulmonary disease said since being diagnosed some parts of his life had become more difficult. 'I miss not being able to play with my grandchildren as much', he said. 'They don't really understand that I just can't do as much now'. Dave, a former smoker of 12 years, said he had his first cigarette at the age of nine. 'The problems I have now are probably due to smoking and working with dangerous substances for work in the past', he said. 'But just because the problems may be from smoking doesn't mean we shouldn't be entitled to support now'.

Extract from the *Gloucester Citizen* newspaper, 'Group eases loneliness of lung disease', 25 August 2006

Figure 8.1 Two newspaper excerpts describing the experiences of people with breast cancer or COPD.

Being able to visualise a disease process mentally and a potential cure affects our attitude to diseases. Most people are extremely apprehensive about cancer and have an image of cancer as something that grows inside the body that could be potentially removed or 'killed' with drugs. Mental metaphors such as those you identified in the newspaper excerpt involve 'fighting' or 'attacking' cancer, and, even if it's unlikely, the patient has the hope that they will be completely cured and returned to their previous, perhaps youthful, vigour. The same is not true of COPD. There is no identifiable disease agency such as a virus infection or tumour cells, so it isn't easy to visualise the cause of the disease. The damage in COPD is widespread, it cannot be removed, and the cause of the damage is probably long departed. There is no cure and the patient will have deteriorated slowly over a long time, so an image of them returning to youthful vigour doesn't come to mind. People with COPD are often depressed and may be withdrawn, anxious and no fun to be with, which may make an onlooker feel helpless and depressed too. There is much less sense of a disease entity as a focus for 'fighting spirit', and therefore less attraction for high-prestige funding and medical research.

People with COPD are often stigmatised in the media, and sometimes by medical professionals, as 'smokers' whose condition is self-inflicted and somehow less worthy of attention. COPD is also perceived to be a condition of old-age or of poorer members of society who have less economic power to attract attention and healthcare funding. Displaying symptoms such as coughing and sputum production may be regarded by other people as annoying or distasteful, which is reflected in the embarrassment many people with COPD feel about coughing in public (Activity 1.1). People with COPD may remain hidden in their homes avoiding social interaction, further reducing public awareness of the condition.

While this may all sound discouraging, recent years have begun to see an increase in the public awareness of COPD through the efforts of global organisations such as WHO and GOLD, local health providers and patient support groups. They have identified that there is a need to educate both the medical community and the general public to recognise the early symptoms of COPD and take action. By 2007, 145 countries, including China but not the USA (Wright and Katz, 2007) had ratified the WHO's tobacco control treaty which aims to regulate tobacco companies by restricting their manufacturing and marketing, raising taxes on tobacco products, limiting smoking in public, and requiring health warnings on cigarette packets. There is also an increasing appreciation that COPD is a treatable condition. Far from just affecting the respiratory system, COPD has consequences for exercise capability, the cardiovascular system, nutritional status and mental health. Approaches such as pulmonary rehabilitation are beginning to address this and are gradually becoming more widely available.

Medical research is also seeking new ways of trying to prevent or even reverse the causative damage to the lungs. As well as improved bronchodilators and anti-inflammatory drugs, one possibility is a drug that inhibits the proteinases that destroy structural proteins such as elastin. Patients who inherit defective alleles of the *AAT* gene and don't have enough active AAT protein to counteract elastase (Box 5.1) can be treated with a weekly infusion of AAT protein that has been extracted from pooled human blood plasma (Stoller and Aboussouan,

2005). Researchers are also exploring the possibilities of gene therapy, in which a defective *AAT* gene allele is replaced with a fully functioning copy. Whether this type of treatment, or drugs that inhibit other types of proteinases, would also be of benefit to other people with COPD is under investigation. The ultimate COPD treatment would be a drug that repairs already damaged lungs. In the late 1990s, scientists discovered that a particular form of vitamin A, which promotes the growth of many tissues in the body, stopped the development of emphysema in animals (Massaro and Massaro, 1997). This looked like an exciting area of research at the time of writing (2007), but only time will tell. There is currently no clear evidence that this treatment is beneficial for human lungs.

COPD has major economic and social costs for societies, but more importantly it affects millions of individuals worldwide by limiting their ability to function, and compromising their quality of life. Until recently, COPD was regarded as the forgotten respiratory disease but there is now a renewed interest in the condition following improvements in diagnosis, and an increasing awareness that it is treatable using a range of measures that address not only prevention and alleviation of symptoms but also its social and psychological impact (Figure 8.2).

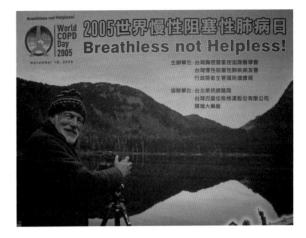

Figure 8.2 World COPD is an annual event promoted by GOLD. World COPD Day poster in Taiwan, with the GOLD slogan: 'Breathless not Helpless!' (Source: European Lung Foundation)

Summary of Chapter 8

8.1 Many individuals with COPD remain undiagnosed and untreated, and public awareness of COPD as a health risk remains low.

8.2 Future hopes for reducing morbidity and mortality from COPD rest on prevention, improved drugs to alleviate symptoms and counter lung damage, and rehabilitation approaches that improve coping skills and exercise tolerance.

Learning outcomes for Chapter 8

After studying this chapter and its associated activities, you should be able to:

LO 8.1 Discuss why the health risk from COPD appears to be so under-appreciated. (Question 8.1)

LO 8.2 Identify the ways in which the management and treatment of COPD may improve in the future. (Question 8.1)

Self-assessment question for Chapter 8

Question 8.1 (LOs 8.1 and 8.2)

How might improving public awareness of COPD reduce morbidity and mortality (Section 1.2) due to this disease?

ANSWERS AND COMMENTS

Answers to self-assessment questions

Question 1.1

COPD is progressive because the irreversible damage caused by exposure to air pollution accumulates and the symptoms gradually worsen. It is a chronic condition because its onset is gradual and its effects are long-lasting.

Question 1.2

In 2030, there are predicted to be 73.25 million deaths from all causes and 5.68 million of these are predicted to be attributable to COPD. To calculate deaths from COPD as a percentage of total deaths, you should have divided 5.68 by 73.25 and multiplied by 100%, so 7.75% of deaths in 2030 are predicted to be attributable to COPD.

Question 2.1

Fewer people may be diagnosed with COPD by a doctor because patients in the early stages may dismiss their symptoms as old age or a 'smoker's cough' and may not seek medical help. Doctors' records of diagnosis may also be hard to interpret because they don't always call the symptoms of COPD by the same name. Spirometry is an objective measure of lung efficiency and diagnosis is made by identifying people with a reduced airflow. People with moderate symptoms who may not yet have felt it necessary to visit a doctor may be included in the diagnosis of COPD.

Question 2.2

There could be many reasons why Africa apparently has a lower COPD prevalence. One likely reason is that Africa has a relatively young population, compared to Europe, so most Africans may not have had a sufficiently long period of exposure to lung-damaging particles. However, you may also have said that perhaps people in Africa overall have a lower exposure to lung-damaging particles from air pollution or tobacco smoking, or that they have less susceptibility to developing COPD because of, for example, inherited genetic factors.

Question 2.3

You may have suggested the following:

Tobacco smoking is a major cause of respiratory diseases including COPD in many countries, particularly those in more affluent industrial regions, for example Europe and the USA, but also increasingly in the newer industrialising regions such as China. Tobacco smoking is prevalent in these regions because of the affordability and availability of tobacco products, but also because of changes in social and cultural attitudes to smoking. In many countries, smoking prevalence has increased because cigarette smoking by women has become increasingly socially acceptable over the last 50 years.

Occupational exposure to dust and smoke particles occurs in many industrial occupations, for example mining, construction, farming and textile production. You may have suggested countries where there are, or have recently been, large mining operations, such as coal mining in the UK or USA. Many industries are now mainly located in areas where cheaper labour is available, for example cotton production in China.

Air pollution from the use of indoor fires or stoves burning coal or biomass fuels is most prevalent in developing countries in regions such as sub-Saharan Africa, and south and central Asia where 'clean' fuels including electricity and gas are less affordable.

Question 3.1

The products of the oxidation of glucose are six molecules of carbon dioxide (CO_2) and six molecules of water (H_2O).

Question 3.2

The partial pressure of nitrogen at sea level is $(78 \div 100) \times 760 = 592.8$ mmHg.

Question 3.3

During expiration the muscles of the ribcage and diaphragm relax, the chest cavity reduces in volume and the natural elasticity of the lungs allows them to recoil, also reducing their volume. The air inside the lungs is compressed, so the gas pressure inside the lungs becomes higher than atmospheric pressure. The air inside the lungs flows out until the pressure inside the lungs equalises with the outside atmospheric pressure.

Question 3.4

Proteins inside the cell don't diffuse out of the cell because they are very large molecules which cannot pass freely through the cell membrane.

Question 4.1

Carbon monoxide binds irreversibly to the same part of haemoglobin as oxygen, the haem, forming carboxyhaemoglobin. Since there will be fewer haemoglobin molecules available to bind oxygen and transport it around in the blood, the tissues of the body will receive less oxygen. The brain cells are particularly sensitive to a lack of oxygen and an individual suffering from severe carbon monoxide poisoning will start to become unconscious as their brain stops functioning.

Question 4.2

Increasing hydrogen ion concentration increases the acidity of a solution which means that it lowers its pH. The pH 5.5 solution would therefore have a higher concentration of hydrogen ions than the pH 7 solution.

Question 4.3

An increased concentration of carbon dioxide in the blood would increase the rate of ventilation by stimulating the respiratory centres in the brain to send a more frequent signal inducing contractions of the muscles of the chest and the diaphragm.

Question 5.1

At a site of injury, damaged cells release inflammatory mediators that cause dilation of the blood vessels so that more blood flows through blood capillaries in the area making it appear red and hot. The walls of the blood capillaries also become leakier, which allows blood plasma to leak out into the tissue causing it to swell.

Question 5.2

The proteinases that damage the lungs in COPD are released by phagocytic cells that are attracted by the inflammatory response. The body tries to counteract the activity of these proteinases by producing a natural proteinase inhibitor called alpha-1 antitrypsin (AAT).

Question 6.1

Both tidal volume (a) and vital capacity (d) expirations can be measured by spirometry, but total lung capacity (b) and residual volume (c) cannot. Residual volume (c) is the volume of air that always remains in the lungs even after a maximum expiration. Since total lung capacity is calculated as the sum of vital capacity (d) and residual volume, it cannot be measured or calculated using spirometry.

Question 6.2

In diagnosis, taking a history of the patient means allowing them to explain their experiences in their own words. From this, a doctor can select information that is relevant to the diagnosis. This is particularly important when diagnosing COPD because some of the symptoms may be similar to those caused by other respiratory problems such as asthma, but the particular circumstances of the individual may point to the correct conclusion. For example, COPD is more likely to be a correct diagnosis if the individual is an older person, and if they have a long history of tobacco smoking or exposure to smoke, dust or fumes.

Question 6.3

You would expect FEV_1 to decrease in both cases. FEV_1 is the volume of air that can be expired in the first second of a forced expiration. It is therefore a good indication of whether there is any kind of obstruction to the airflow out of the lungs. During an asthma attack, the muscles in the walls of the airways temporarily constrict, narrowing the airways and creating an obstruction to airflow, so FEV_1 would be lower than the predicted level for a person with healthy lungs. In COPD, airflow is also obstructed by permanent narrowing of the airways and loss of elastic recoil of the lungs preventing efficient expiration. FEV_1 would therefore also be lower in COPD.

Question 7.1

First, relievers help to reduce narrowing of the airways by relaxing the smooth muscles that form bands around the larger airways. In some COPD patients, this helps to open up the airways improving the airflow through lungs and reducing breathlessness, especially if the drug is inhaled before exercise. Second, opening up the airways can also help to expel mucus. These drugs sometimes have little effect because the narrowing of airways in COPD may be due to an irreversible thickening of the walls of the airways by the swelling associated with inflammation and the laying down of scar tissues.

Question 7.2

For people with COPD, physical effort brings on breathlessness and fatigue, so to reduce their symptoms many people abandon normal activities such as working, sport and socialising. This will inevitably reduce their social interaction with other people. People may also find it difficult to socialise because of their embarrassment about coughing, or appearing ill or weak in public. They may also go out less because they worry about having exacerbations or panic attacks when they are away from home. Anxiety and depression likewise tend to lead to social withdrawal.

Question 8.1

Increasing public awareness of COPD may ensure that more people seek help at an earlier stage where prevention and treatment would be more effective. More awareness about COPD may also ensure that demand for appropriate treatments makes resources more widely available.

Comments on activities

Activity 2.1

We identified the following measures that could reduce the health effects of indoor smoke on Nadira's family; you may have thought of others:

- Installing a hood or chimney above the cooking fire to draw out the smoke.
- Installing an improved cooking stove ventilated by a flue to remove smoke and confine the fuel in a smaller space making it burn more efficiently producing less smoke.
- Providing access to cleaner liquid or gaseous fuels that don't produce smoke or dust.
- Reducing heating requirements by installing insulation or solar power heating.
- Cooking outdoors or in open cooking shelters.
- Improving ventilation, e.g. increasing the number of windows or providing gaps between the roof and walls.
- Education about the risks of exposure to cooking smoke, e.g. encouraging mothers to keep their young babies and children away from the fire.

We identified the following difficulties that may be encountered in enabling, or persuading the family to take up these measures:

- Poorer households may not be able to afford to use more expensive cleaner fuels.

- Where there isn't a large market for improved cooking stoves and cleaner sources of energy, many rural communities don't develop the resources to make or supply them.

- Improving the ventilation may also make the house colder. People often seal up holes to prevent drafts, or to keep insects out.

- Families may have social and cultural objections to changes in their lifestyle, particularly if they are imposed by outsiders.

- Families may be used to preparing food in particular ways, or they may have difficulty learning to use a new stove design.

Activity 6.1

1   The flow–volume curve angles inward on the way down because in emphysema the floppy airways tend to collapse near the end of the expiration, slowing down the rate of airflow even more so that the slope becomes shallower.

2   There is no change in the shape of the flow–volume curve representing this patient's airflow after she has been treated with a bronchodilator. This indicates that she is likely to have COPD and not asthma. She may not get much relief from regular treatment with bronchodilator drugs.

3   The carbon monoxide molecules inspired during the gas transfer test bind tightly to haemoglobin in the red blood cells and are carried away in the blood circulation.

Activity 7.1

We identified the following concerns expressed by the Breazers in Activity 1.1 that are also reflected in the USA survey:

- The frustration of not being able to plan ahead (e.g. shopping trips) because things are frequently disrupted by an exacerbation. Life is put on hold temporarily because the person can't do anything except rest, and often doesn't want to be in the company of others.

- Not being able to do normal chores such as making the bed.

- Not being able to walk, and having to rely on transport, even for the shortest trips.

- The feeling they 'can't enjoy themselves any more' because they've had to give up life-long recreational pursuits such as gardening or dancing.

- The embarrassment of coughing, which prevents social activities such as going to the theatre, as well as a sense of hurt at the disapproving attitude of other people.

Activity 7.2

As well as improving fitness and exercise tolerance, these sessions help to reduce the anxiety that getting breathless will be harmful. This gives the participants the confidence to continue with normal physical activities such as walking and exercising, so that they can lead as normal a life as possible and prevent the cycle of decline due to inactivity. There is also a wide range of advice available for many aspects of lifestyle, not just medication. The supervisors of the session encourage an element of competition and there is certainly a sense of achievement that motivates the participants to continue to exercise. Any sense of isolation is also reduced by seeing other people with similar problems learning to cope. This is reflected in the friendly atmosphere of the Breazers group (Activity 1.1) where the members can socialise without having to be embarrassed about coughing or breathing difficulties.

References and Further reading

References

Ambrosino, N. and Simonds, A. (2007) 'The clinical management in extremely severe COPD', *Respiratory Medicine*, vol. 101, pp. 1613–1624.

Anthonisen, N. R., Connet, J. E. and Murray, R. P. (2002) 'Smoking and lung function of Lung Health Study participants after 11 years', *American Journal of Respiratory and Critical Care Medicine*, vol. 166, pp. 675–679.

Berger, B. G., and Motl, R. W. (2000) 'Exercise and mood: A selective review and synthesis of research employing the profile of mood states', *Journal of Applied Sports Psychology*, vol. 12, pp. 69–92.

Boschetto, P., Quintavalle, S., Miotto, D., Lo Cascio, N., Zeni, E. and Mapp, C. E. (2006) 'Chronic obstructive pulmonary disease (COPD) and occupational exposures', *Journal of Occupational Medicine and Toxicology*, vol. 1, p. 11.

Bruce, N., Perez-Padilla, R. and Albalak, R. (2002) 'Indoor air pollution in developing countries: a major environmental and public health challenge', *Bulletin of the World Health Organization*, vol. 78, pp. 1078–1092.

Celli, B. R. (2006) 'Chronic obstructive pulmonary disease: from unjustified nihilism to evidence-based optimism', *Proceedings of the American Thoracic Society*, vol. 3, pp. 58–65.

Chapman, R. S., He, X., Blair, A. E. and Lan, Q. (2005) 'Improvement in household stoves and risk of chronic obstructive pulmonary disease in Xuanwei, China: retrospective cohort study', *British Medical Journal*, vol. 331, p. 1050.

Currie, G. P. and Douglas, J. G. (2006) 'Oxygen and inhalers', *British Medical Journal*, vol. 333, pp. 34–36.

Currie, G. P. and Legge, J. S. (2006) 'ABC of chronic obstructive pulmonary disease. Diagnosis', *British Medical Journal*, vol. 332, pp. 1261–1263.

de Marco, R., Accordini, S., Cerveri, I., Corsico, A., Sunyer, J., Neukirch, F., Kunzli, N., Leynaert, B., Janson, C., Gislason, T., Vermeire, P., Svanes, C., Anto, J. M. and Burney, P. (2004) European Community Respiratory Health Survey Study Group. An international survey of chronic obstructive pulmonary disease in young adults according to GOLD stages. *Thorax*, vol. 59, pp. 120–125.

Dowson, C., Laing, R., Barraclough, R., Town, I., Mulder, R., Norris, K. and Drennan, C. (2001) 'The use of the Hospital Anxiety and Depression Scale (HADS) in patients with chronic obstructive pulmonary disease: a pilot study', *New Zealand Medical Journal*, vol. 114, pp. 447–449.

Ekici, A., Ekici, M., Kurtipek, E., Akin, A., Arslan, M., Kara, T., Apaydin, Z. and Demir, S. (2005) 'Obstructive airway diseases in women exposed to biomass smoke', *Environmental Research*, vol. 99, pp. 93–98.

Fletcher, C. and Peto, R. (1977) 'The natural history of chronic airflow obstruction', *British Medical Journal*, vol. 1, pp. 1645–1648.

Halbert, R. J., Isonaka, S., George, D. and Iqbal, A. (2003) 'Interpreting COPD prevalence estimates: what is the true burden of disease?', *Chest*, vol. 123, pp. 1684–1692.

Halliday, T. R. and Davey, G. C. B. (eds) (2007) *Water and Health in an Overcrowded World*, Oxford, Oxford University Press.

Hnizdo, E., Sullivan, P. A., Bang, K. M. and Wagner, G. (2002) 'Association between chronic obstructive pulmonary disease and employment by industry and occupation in the US population: a study of data from the Third National Health and Nutrition Examination Survey', *American Journal of Epidemiology*, vol. 156, pp. 738–746.

Jeffery, P. K. (2000) 'Comparison of the structural and inflammatory features of COPD and asthma', Giles F. Filley Lecture, *Chest*, vol. 117, pp. 251S–260S.

Kazerouni, N., Alverson, C. J., Redd, S. C., Mott, J. A. and Mannino, D. M. (2004) 'Sex differences in COPD and lung cancer mortality trends – United States', 1968–1999. (2004) *Journal of Women's Health*, vol. 13, pp. 17–23.

Kikawada, M., Ichinose, Y., Miyamoto, D., Minemura, K., Takasaki, M. and Toyama, K. (2000) 'Peripheral airway findings in chronic obstructive pulmonary disease using an ultrathin bronchoscope', *The European Respiratory Journal*, vol. 15, pp. 105–108.

Knudson, R. J., Slatin, R. C., Lewowitz, M. D. and Burrows, B. (1976) 'The maximal expiratory flow-volume curve: normal standards variability, and effect of age'. *American Review of Respiratory Disease*, vol. 113, pp. 587–600.

Lacasse, Y., Goldstein, R., Lasserson, T. J. and Martin, S. (2006) 'Pulmonary rehabilitation for chronic obstructive pulmonary disease', *Cochrane Database of Systematic Reviews* [online], Issue 4, Article No. CD003793.

Løkke, A., Lange, P., Scharling, H., Fabricius, P. and Vestbo, J. (2006) 'Developing COPD: a 25 year follow up study of the general population', *Thorax*, vol. 61, pp. 935–939.

Lyubomirsky, S., Sheldon, K. M. and Schkade, D. (2005). 'Pursuing happiness: the architecture of sustainable change', *Review of General Psychology*, vol. 9, pp. 111–131.

Mackay, J., Eriksen, M. and Shafey, O. (2006) *The Tobacco Atlas*, 2nd edn, Atlanta, American Cancer Society.

Mannino, D. M. (2002) 'COPD: epidemiology, prevalence, morbidity and mortality, and disease heterogeneity', *Chest*, vol. 121, pp. 121S–126S.

Massaro, G. D. and Massaro, D. (1997) 'Retinoic acid treatment abrogates elastase-induced pulmonary emphysema in rats', *Nature Medicine*, vol. 3, pp. 675–677.

Mathers, C. D. and Loncar, D. (2006) 'Projections of global mortality and burden of disease from 2002 to 2030', *PLoS Medicine*, vol. 3, p. 442.

McLannahan, H. (ed.) (2008) *Visual Impairment: A Global View*, Oxford, Oxford University Press, in press.

Menezes, A. M., Perez-Padilla, R., Jardim, J. R, Muino, A., Lopez, M. V., Valdivia, G., Montes de Oca, M., Talamo, C., Hallal, P. C. and Victora, C. G (2005) 'Chronic obstructive pulmonary disease in five Latin American cities (the PLATINO study): a prevalence study', *The Lancet*, vol. 366, pp. 1875–1881.

Menezes, A. M. B. and Victora, C. G. (2005) Report presented by the Chile Platino Study Team: Platino Study – Chilean survey, Federal University of Pelotas, Brazil.

Murray, C. J. L. and Lopez, A. D. (1997) 'Mortality by cause for eight regions of the world: Global Burden of Disease study', *The Lancet*, vol. 349, pp. 1269–1276.

Needham, M. and Stockley, R. A. (2004) 'Alpha-1 antitrypsin deficiency. 3: clinical manifestations and natural history', *Thorax*, vol. 59, pp. 441–445.

Parvin, E. M. (ed.) (2007) *Screening for Breast Cancer*, Oxford, Oxford University Press.

Phillips, J. B. (ed.) (2008) *Trauma, Repair and Recovery*, Oxford, Oxford University Press, in press.

Pokhrel, A. K., Smith, K. R, Khalakdina, A., Deuja, A. and Bates, M. N. (2005) 'Case-control study of indoor cooking smoke exposure and cataract in Nepal and India', *International Journal of Epidemiology*, vol. 34, pp. 702–708.

Prescott, E. and Vestbo, J. (1999) 'Socioeconomic status and chronic obstructive pulmonary disease', *Thorax*, vol. 54, pp. 737–741.

Ram, F. S., Rodriguez-Roisin, R., Granados-Navarrete, A., Garcia-Aymerich, J. and Barnes, N. C. (2006) 'Antibiotics for exacerbations of chronic obstructive pulmonary disease', *Cochrane Database of Systematic Reviews* [online], Issue 2. Article No. CD004403.

Rodgers., A., Ezzati, M., Vander Hoorn, S., Lopez, A. D., Lin, R-B. and Murray, C. J. L. (2004) 'Distribution of major health risks: findings from the global burden of disease study', *PLoS Medicine*, vol. 1, pp. 44–55.

Schulman, Ronca and Bucuvalas Inc. (2001) Confronting COPD in North America and Europe: A survey of patients and doctors in eight countries. Executive summary. Available at: http://www.copdinamerica.com (Accessed April 2007)

Shrestha, I. L. and Shrestha, S. L. (2005) 'Indoor air pollution from biomass fuels and respiratory health of the exposed population in Nepalese households', *International Journal of Occupational and Environmental Health*, vol. 11, pp. 150–160.

Smart, L. E. (ed.) (2007) *Alcohol and Human Health*, Oxford, Oxford University Press.

Smith, K. R., Samet, J. M., Romieu, I. and Bruce, N. (2000) Indoor air pollution in developing countries and acute lower respiratory infections in children. *Thorax*, vol. 55, pp. 518–532.

Stoller, J. K. and Aboussouan, L. S. (2005) 'Alpha-1 antitrypsin deficiency', *The Lancet*, vol. 365, pp. 2225–2236.

Toates, F. (ed.) (2007) *Pain*, Oxford, Oxford University Press.

van Ede, L., Yzermans, C. J. and Brouwer, H. J. (1999) 'Prevalence of depression in patients with chronic obstructive pulmonary disease: a systematic review', *Thorax*, vol. 54, pp. 688–692.

Warwick, H. and Doig, A. (2004) *Smoke – the Killer in the Kitchen*, London, ITDG Publishing.

WHO (2002a) *World Health Report 2002: Reducing Risks, Promoting Healthy Life*, Geneva, World Health Organization.

WHO (2002b) *The Global Burden of Disease Study, 2002*, Geneva, World Health Organization.

WHO (2006) *World Health Report 2006: Working Together for Health*, Geneva, World Health Organization.

Wright, A. A. and Katz, I. T. (2007) 'Tobacco tightrope – balancing disease prevention and economic development in China', *New England Journal of Medicine*, vol. 356, pp. 1493–1496.

Zhang, H. and Cai, B. (2003) 'The impact of tobacco on lung health in China', *Respirology*, vol. 8, pp. 17–21.

Further reading

Halpin, D. M. G. (2003) *COPD: Your Questions Answered*, London, Churchill Livingstone.

Hansel, T. T. and Barnes, P. J. (2003) *An Atlas of Chronic Obstructive Pulmonary Disease* (Encyclopaedia of Visual Medicine Series), London, New York, Parthenon Publishing.

Useful websites, maintained by the OU Library through the ROUTES system (see 'About this book')

British Lung Foundation

http://www.lunguk.org/copd.asp [This website has information for people with COPD, and links to information about the activities of this organisation which supports people with different types of lung disease.]

World Health Organization

http://www.who.int/respiratory/copd/en/ [This website links to information about the impact of COPD globally.]

PatientPlus

http://www.patient.co.uk/showdoc/40000625/ [This website has information for people with COPD and links to other sources of information and support in the UK.]

ACKNOWLEDGEMENTS

Grateful acknowledgement is made to the following sources for permission to reproduce material in this book.

Figure 1.1: Karen Robinson/Panos Pictures; Figure 1.3: Carol Midgley;

Figure 2.1: WHO/Global Burden of Disease Study; Figure 2.3: Kazerouni, N. et al. (2004) 'Sex differences in COPD and lung cancer mortality trends – United States, 1968–1999', *Journal of Womens Health*, vol. 13 (1) © Mary Anne Liebert Inc; Figure 2.4: Image courtesy of The Advertising Archives; Figure 2.5: Adapted from Mackay, J. et al. (2006) *The Tobacco Atlas* (2nd edn), American Cancer Society; Figure 2.6: Arturo Delfin/Morguefile; Figure 2.7: China Photos/Getty Images; Figures 2.8 and 2.10: Warwick, H. and Doig, A. (2004) *Smoke – the Killer in the Kitchen*, ITDG Publishing; Figures 2.9 and 2.11 Alex Duncan; Figure 2.12: Chapman, R. S. et al. (2005) 'Improvement in household stoves and risk of chronic obstructive pulmonary disease in Zuanwei', *British Medical Journal*, vol. 331, British Medical Association; Figure 2.13: Getty Images; Figure 2.14: PA Photos;

Figure 3.1: Mike Levers/Open University; Figure 3.4: Susumu Nishinaga/Science Photo Library; Figure 3.5: Dr. Walter Weder (Institute of Anatomy, University of Bern, Bern, Switzerland);

Figure 5.3: Arnold Brody/Science Photo Library; Figure 5.4a, b: Wellcome Institute Library Photographic Library; Figure 5.4c, d: Jeffery, P. K. (2000) 'Comparison of the structural and inflammatory features of COPD and Asthma', *Chest*, vol. 117, May, American College of Chest Physicians; Figure 5.4d, e: Kikawada, M. et al. (2000) 'Peripheral airway findings in chronic obstructive pulmonary disease using an ultrathin bronchoscope', *European Respiratory Journal*, vol. 15, ERS Journals Ltd;

Figure 6.1a: GJLP/CNRI/Science Photo Library; Figure 6.1b: Du Cane Medical Imaging Ltd/Science Photo Library;

Figures 7.1, 7.2 and 7.3: Confronting COPD in America survey, 2001, conducted by SRBI and funded by GlaxoSmithKline;

Figure 8.1: Symons, J. (2005) 'Patient power – what to do if you're in a row with the NHS', *The Sun*, 3 November and (2006) 'Group eases loneliness of lung disease', *Gloucester Citizen*, 25 August; Figure 8.2: European Lung Foundation.

Every effort has been made to contact copyright holders. If any have been inadvertently overlooked the publishers will be pleased to make the necessary arrangements at the first opportunity.

INDEX

Entries and page numbers in **bold type** refer to key words which are printed in **bold** in the text. Indexed information on pages indicated by *italics* is carried mainly or wholly in a figure or a table.